THE SOUL OF THE NURSE

THE SOUL OF THE NURSE

ELIZABETH ANN ROBINSON, PHD, RN, CNS

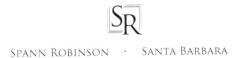

SPANN ROBINSON · SANTA BARBARA

Robinson, Elizabeth Ann.
  The Soul of the Nurse

  ISBN-13: 978-1480284241
  ISBN-10: 1480284246
  Library of Congress Control Number: 2012922098

First Edition, 2013.
Printed in the United States of America

For Bibliography, visit: www.SpannRobinson.com

Cover and book design: SpannRobinson and Lyza Fontana
Photo of the author: Jill Martin, www.kindeyes.com
Cover photo: Tracie Walker and Kathy Morison
              The Nurses Memorial at Arlington National Cemetery

For book ordering information and permission to reproduce selections,
please contact:

Spann Robinson
735 State Street
Suite 628
Santa Barbara, California 93101
SpannRobinson@gmail.com

www.SpannRobinson.com

SpannRobinson is dedicated to literature, writing, healthcare,
mythology, archetypal psychology, body awareness, and imagination.
Lawrence Henry Spann and Elizabeth Ann Robinson write and edit
their own books. For more information about events, workshops, and
book releases, please visit the website.

Thank you, Lawrence Henry Spann
*Your love for authentic voice and your editorial
rigor have made this book possible.*

Dedication
*For the nurse, past, present, and future.
I remain in awe.*

TABLE OF CONTENTS

INTRODUCTION

When I started talking about the nurse as the subject for this book I was amazed at how many people were interested—nurses and non-nurses alike. Not only does the nurse captivate culture, consciously and unconsciously, but she is someone everyone knows from experience as a patient, visitor, relative, or friend. I love the nurse—what she is capable of, her resilience, and no nonsense approach to the most bizarre, disconcerting, and unpredictable experiences in her everyday work. Rather than running away from emergencies, the nurse runs towards them.

Year after year, Gallup polls show that the public holds the nurse as the most trusted professional in society, her honesty and ethical standards consistently rated "very high" or "high," well above physicians, police officers, and chaplains. The professional nurse is the backbone of healthcare. She is the most important reason patients need to be in the hospital, and clearly hospitals cannot function without them. As a nurse, I've worked in oncology, cardiology, and critical care in major university medical centers and community hospitals. As a Clinical Nurse Specialist (CNS), I have supported nurses of all kinds, and, as a patient, I've personally experienced a variety of nurses directly caring for me.

THE SOUL OF THE NURSE

While pursuing doctoral studies, I found nursing programs too narrowly focused and limited to a specific area of study. I had always been drawn to Jungian psychology and had never taken time to study the humanities. So, when I found one school in the country that offered a PhD in Mythological Studies with Emphasis in Depth Psychology, I jumped at the opportunity to go. This approach to the humanities, combined with my science background and experience as a nurse and a patient, yielded the book you are about to read.

Since historically nurses have almost always been women, and today 95% are women, *The Soul of the Nurse* is written from the perspective of the nurse living in a female body. This does not exclude men but orients the nurse and her function from the feminine perspective, which, in the setting of this vocation, applies to men as well. It is compassion, eros, openness to body and instincts, and a more circular and tragic sensibility that dominates the earliest archetypal patterns of the nurse. And if we are to begin to understand the nurse mythologically we must unravel her link to womanhood.

The archetype of the nurse lives in me differently than it does in other nurses; thus some of my findings will not resonate with everyone. It is up to each nurse to explore the

INTRODUCTION

images and stories that resonate for her because mythological and archetypal awareness can deepen her connection to the true origins of the nurse. Fully developed feminine strength is desperately needed today in full partnership with our masculine-dominated healthcare system.

Mythologically, the nurse is the guide to souls, like the Greek mythic figure, Hecate. She is able to perceive what others cannot. So perceptive to when others are in danger, Hecate is the only one who heard Persephone scream as she was dragged into the underworld. She bears witness to other people's lives when the boundary between life and death is uncertain. Hecate can relate to wild and dark emotions because she has learned from her own abandonment and suffering how to be present with others in their suffering. No matter the era, the archetype of the nurse is compelling.

Nursing today is practiced in a fractured and business-like environment, operating for profit with quick fixes to increase cash flow. The forces of insurance, consumerism, the drug and device industry, media, advertising, and the legal community have greatly impacted nursing practice. In the past, like Hecate, the nurse approached the whole person. Today, nurses search for soul in a dry corporate environment where the true soul of the nurse is dismissed and disregarded.

As I explored the origins of the nurse in mythology, archeology, fairy tales, art, literature, television, and film, I began to understand how the nurse image has been split into pieces—or dismembered. I found that the nurse archetype cannot be accessed through reason alone. It became clear that an imaginative approach was necessary.

The needle is associated with the nurse literally and symbolically. We all remember the nurse giving us shots as youngsters. The needle is also connected to many indigenous rituals that require sharp objects to ward off evil spirits. Needles can make one fall asleep, die, or recover. In suturing, a needle and thread joins tissue together. I will use personal stories as threads to join my myth with collective myths throughout this book.

Why did I become a nurse? This is the first question every nurse might ask herself. My reason became clear as I integrated the material while writing this book. I was certainly never encouraged to be a nurse and there were no nurses in my family other than my grandmother's estranged sister, Great Aunt Gladys, whom I never met, even though she lived well into my adulthood. After my grandmother died, I found a small formal black and white photo of Gladys proudly wearing a nurse's cap and uniform. Gladys is buried, near eight of my maternal ancestors, in a cemetery overlooking the Pacific Ocean where I now live. All I ever heard about Gladys was that she'd show up at family gatherings in a convertible with a new man in tow. Sounds like a lot of fun to me. I truly wish I'd known her.

After the death of my parents and dissolution of ties with my brothers and the paternal family ranch in central California, I moved to this new place so heavily infused with my feminine roots. Through immersion in mythology, I realized I did not have to be the literal sacrificed daughter; I could call on Iphigenia. I no longer had to live the role of dutiful daughter; I could call on Cordelia and Antigone. And I did not have to live out the fate of the martyred visionary; I could call on Cassandra. Just as the archetypal mother is much more powerful than the personal mother, archetypal figures are always stronger than any of the personal figures in our lives. They continue to show me I am not alone.

Each life is a search for its own personal mythology. We as nurses share common rituals and links to ancient stories. At the deepest level, each of us locates our personal destiny through the collective myths that have seeped like water through porous bedrock for thousands of years.

THE SOUL OF THE NURSE

The healthcare system is in deep need of these life-giving waters.

CHAPTER 1
The Nurse

The soul stirs and draws the nurse to her profession. At the core is a call and a sense of mission. The origin of nursing as a religious vocation is only part of the story. It does not answer the deeper question because vocation also relates to voice, as in giving voice to an inner calling, one that evokes strong feelings through memory and imagination. A calling is primal—a heart-felt inner knowing directed at one's personal destiny. Some nurses do not feel this calling but are talked into it. Some make the decision for financial reasons or because shift work offers a practical way to earn a living with flexibility. Most find, once they are inside the profession, it is a calling. Those who do not experience this have a difficult time maintaining their professional livelihood.

While the public trusts the nurse more than any other professional, they also idealize or denigrate her image, often making her into a one-dimensional caricature or stereotype. Nurses accept these labels and disguises. Throughout the book I use these stereotypes as a starting place. For example, symbolically the nurse image holds the opposites of angel and witch without judgment. This is important because black and white thinking limits imagination. It is important not to reject a limited image because considering all the pieces is necessary in order to re-member the nurse in all her depth and complexity. Each split-off image has something to say about the whole.

The profession of nursing was founded on silence. Today the nurse needs to develop a strong authentic voice to meet the calling of her vocation. Often the calling to serve the wounded originates from an unconscious desire to address personal suffering—the wounded-healer motif. The nurse knows, at least on an unconscious level, that the effects of true healing go both ways. United, the nurse communicates with the patient somewhere between soul and spirit with rituals directed to the body. She experiences nuances, openings, a shift of the body, or an expression, all while maintaining presence with the vulnerable patient.

There is a bond of loyalty and responsibility between nurse and patient. More importantly there is mystery and depth beyond words. When that's missing, the relationship is simply mechanical, cold, and lonely. The nurse-patient relationship is difficult to describe in concrete terms but, as any nurse or caretaker knows, at times it feels numinous. The togetherness is complex and not rational, thus inexplicable. Nurses know that within this bond the potential for transformation is extraordinary, yet only on rare occasions do nurses speak about it to others.

During an intense time of potential transformation, it is the nurse who provides basic and advanced care while translating medical jargon, supporting, and validating the patient. The nurse who cultivates skill, knowledge, and caring is the most competent and effective nurse. In a fragmented healthcare system, the nurse can easily be side-tracked and forget that love and caring are primal needs.

In addition to the highly skilled and challenging intellectual work, the nurse also does many mundane tasks. She makes beds, gives baths, all while assessing every bruise, abrasion, and beginning of a bed sore. She feeds, gives cool and hot washcloths, holds emesis basins, and cleans up incontinent stool, urine, and other body secretions, all while sensitized to and aware of body parts, sounds, and subtleties—an intimacy not known to any other profession. For the nurse, spirit resides in matter and the sacred is found in the profane. The physical proximity creates, out of necessity, endless potential for layers of deep communication between patient and nurse.

Women have assumed the role of nurse since the beginning of time. Family members and slaves were enrolled as caregivers.

Mythological figures like Hygeia and Panacea, in ancient Greece, set the stage for silenced and invisible women—like nuns, deaconesses, matrons, spinsters, and other women—who cared for the sick. Nurses of biblical times symbolize duty as servant, companion, and helpmate.

Historically the nurse wears a veil, a habit, a cap, a cape: a uniform. She is ascetic, self-abnegating, and obedient. She has religious, military, and puritanical roots. During the Inquisition women who offered practical nursing and health remedies were deemed witches and executed. Males served as nurses during the Crusades. Pope Innocent VIII's 1484 decree, used for three centuries, explains how to investigate, interrogate, and execute witches, claiming all women are potential witches due to their insatiable lust, slippery tongues, weakness, and association with devils. No wonder nurses today hide their true powers and secret skills.

In 1843, British novelist, Charles Dickens, accurately portrayed the nurse of his times in the character of Sarah Gamp, an unsophisticated, vulgar, slovenly drunk and criminal. Modern nursing wasn't formalized until the mid-19th century when Florence Nightingale established it as a respected profession.

Rules of behavior that have favored the masculine perspective for thousands of years have left nurses wounded on a personal and collective level. Wounds from societal norms as well as parents or partners can create what feels like being invisible, or non-existent, which might help explain the chronic invisibility of nurses. When the profession cannot carry the flame, each nurse must find her own.

Nurse as Mythologist

Mythology and folklore offer an unparalleled opportunity for exploring unconscious material. As I moved into collective stories, I discovered universal archetypal patterns. This naturally required dismembering assumptions deeply imbedded in my personal, ancestral, and cultural psyche. It was through this movement back and forth, between the personal and collective, that insights were revealed. By exploring the various nurse figures found in mythology, fairy tales, and other narratives, I found clues into what's really going on beneath the surface as these stories resonated with my own experience.

Archetypes, although formless, are felt in the body and perceived as images in the mind. Many of these symbolic representations reverberated in my whole being. This will become apparent as you read on. I learned to tolerate paradox—two extremes that seem contradictory. I found that it enriched and energized my experience. Imagination brought meaning to the instinctual feelings that had a natural link between my female body and mind. I learned that archetypes cannot be explained, only experienced, and only within each of our own personal and cultural biases. For example, I was particularly drawn to nurse figures from Western traditions.

It is important to understand that we can never grasp an archetype per se but can begin to get glimpses of archetypes through the way they influence human behavior and how they appear in world myths. Archetypes never go away but sometimes go underground and seem hidden. A good rule of thumb is, when you feel drawn in and repelled at the same time, you have entered an archetype. An archetype holds both light and dark, creative and destructive, disturbing and appealing—it always contains contradictions which make us uncomfortable. There is energy created by ambivalence, which is why an archetype is expansive. When we deny, moralize, and sort the good from the bad, some of the dynamic vitality of the image is lost. Repressed content always makes itself known in other ways.

If we deny the nurse as angel, we are deprived of her altruism, or if we disavow the nurse as witch, we lose her intuition and perception. If we reject the nurse as erotic, we dismiss her comfort with tending a stranger's body, and, if we refuse to admit the sacrificial servant, we forget her ability to tend to others' needs first. If we dismiss the strict matron, we disregard her vigilance and the rage that feeds her ability to protect the vulnerable. And, of course, all of these are the core aspects of who the nurse really is.

Without this shift from an unconscious, reactionary place, one remains stuck in linear thinking. Eros, longing, and a heartfelt orientation are more in tune with the true nature of the nurse. Eros seeks not perfection but unity, relatedness, and connection to the body and instincts. Reactionary power seeks perfection. I learned through mythology that perfection is for gods and goddesses, not human beings. Eros opens body and soul to what matters. The connection between instinct and image brings union. It is eros that moves us to embrace soul, moving away from power, materialism, and the unreachable ideal of perfection. At the core of symbolic representations of the nurse is a powerful mystery.

Becoming a separate, more fully evolved individual requires ongoing interaction between the superficial and deeper facets of our being, which is often uncomfortable. It demands diving into particulars that have been repressed, eliciting both pleasure and pain. Facing illusion is difficult. Since personal growth and self-care are not supported in most healthcare settings, it makes inner work for each nurse a solo journey. Inner work is about penetrating pathos, going in, down, and back in order to become aware of one's personal realities and illusions. Only when each nurse does her inner work can there be a real impact on the nursing profession.

Inner Work

The nurse is drawn by her very nature to paradox. Things are often the opposite of what they seem. In order to flourish the nurse must open to something greater than herself, connect to her inner core and retrieve the sacredness of service that prompted her to become a nurse in the first place. This involves a re-imagining, unconstrained by dogma and known practices, retrieving inner knowing, rejecting ideologies— essentially following her true path.

The ancient Greeks embraced a broad spectrum of life as revealed in their divinities. Mythology diversifies ways to explore concepts buried in the unconscious. By approaching the individual and the collective with curiosity and self-acceptance, the nurse finds more possibility for affirmation among colleagues and therefore better relationships. Getting in touch with herself makes each nurse a better nurse.

THE NURSE

Nurses are resilient and subject to rigorous work with constant exposure to the ambiguous nature of the profession. A conscious awareness of paradox paves the way to wisdom and a thriving practice. Embracing paradox enables the nurse to experience each of her daily encounters and rituals in a more profound way.

Midwife for End of Life

We fear endings in our culture and there is tremendous confusion around the end of life. What the patient wants, what is realistic, and what constitutes compassionate care often do not match. Heroics that save many lives can also prolong suffering. Since most people are inexperienced and unprepared to make decisions about end-of-life care, there is often little choice offered but to continue artificial life support measures. The nurse is left to attend the patient with few tools to ease the agony other than sedatives and narcotics. I have never met a nurse uncomfortable with allowing natural death at the end of life. It is a ritual and the nurse is ritual leader in a sacred art learned over time.

Decisions about end of life are not and should not be easy. There is no ideology here, just hard work. There are consequences in each action. Preservation of life and allowing natural death both require keeping relationships intact. The complexity of each decision must be carefully considered. For the nurse, birth and death are opposite ends of the spectrum. Family, visitors, and physicians come and go while nurses remain throughout the 24 hour reality. The nurse is witness on a moment to moment basis.

It is important to the nurse that the patient not die alone. Even in the early days before modern nursing, a "watcher" would sit with a dying patient. When a patient dies, the nurse continues her care with the post-mortem ritual which lessens some of the obvious signs of suffering. She cleans the body and tidies the room. She presents the body for loved ones to view and touch. This ritual ends when the nurse transfers the body to the gurney that carries it to the morgue. Only then is her responsibility relinquished.

Unfortunately, in most cases the funeral industry, not the loved ones, take control from there. For over a hundred years we have handed over our dead to strangers. Perhaps the death ritual is a symptom of the loss of soul in general. It seems our material focus has translated to people. Morticians restore the body which does little to change the fact that the body will decay in a coffin or be cremated. Restoration and embalming represent a flawed attempt to cope with loss, anxiety, and confusion. It is easy to fall into the funeral industry's ideology and trivialities in an attempt to repress grief and mourning. The soul's way is not of simplicity but of complexity. Since the soul has a deep desire to mourn, we need a new mythos around death that is shared by the community.

Illness Speaks for Soul

We are all patients, and nurses have all experienced being ill. Paradoxically, physical illness can be, as Freud referred to dreams, "the royal road to the unconscious," or it can have no meaning at all. Myth and dream come from the wisdom of the body. The nurse knows that her patient's illness can provide an unparalleled chance to acknowledge a hidden message. Vulnerability creates an openness to face questions about life's purpose and destiny. Information is liberated from the unconscious through illness in the form of a message from the soul.

Nurses are constantly faced with trauma. The nurse, like the therapist, is comfortable in the underworld. She has an ability to handle crisis and drama likely because of the way in which she was raised. The setting feels comfortable and she can find a place for herself in the system. Yet we know that there is a limit to how much trauma anyone can take. When the emotional experience becomes too much, her psyche learns to split off parts, leaving her with an empty feeling, loss of meaning, and ultimately an inability to experience life in its fullness.

I've often wondered about the nurse and her own inner patient. As a patient, I have always known when it is time for further investigation or biopsies, even when physicians assured me that the symptom was nothing. When I was sixteen I looked and felt like I was in great health, busy with swimming, playing water polo, and diving. I found a lump above my right clavicle and asked my father to take me to see our family physician. The physician wanted to watch it for a few weeks. At that point, I insisted on a biopsy. My little hometown pathology department could not, or would not, make the diagnosis and sent the specimen to Stanford, who called immediately reporting Hodgkin's Disease, cancer of the lymphatic system. My mother and I set out for Stanford the same day.

During this experience, I encountered my inner patient. I nursed and found compassion for myself I didn't know existed. As a child, I always needed time alone to be with my feelings, so I embraced my melancholy which I intuitively knew was important. This allowed for a slowing down to the essentials as I began contemplating life, death, love, the greater power of divinity, and friendship. Colors, sounds, smells, and nature became more vivid. The character of people around me grew important as new friends emerged and old friends became distant. Little annoyances fell away, and what was truly important became large and loud. Little acts of kindness and mannerisms of healthcare practitioners and strangers seemed huge now as I faced new limitations and new passions within my inescapable disease. I began to hear and see and absorb everything more sensitively.

Near Stanford I stayed with my parents' friend, Barbara Peterson, who became a wise elder. She coached me before each radiation treatment not to resist the rays but to welcome them into my body. She taught me to visualize the radiation destroying only the cancer cells and preserving the healthy cells. She had a huge pitcher of water waiting for me when I returned from treatment. She said to visualize the water washing the cancer cells out.

Modern medicine stifles the experience of illness by making it purely physical with no regard to its role as bearer of information. The patient is not approached as partner. Illness is seen as an enemy to be fought with every possible means. Hospitals are battlefields where we fight rather than listen and cooperate with disease. The use of statements like "lost his fight with cancer" or "made a valiant effort in her battle against cancer" dismisses the fact that illness is part of the human experience. Modern medicine's thirst for power and "battle" with illness reveals the sad fact that medicine suppresses the humanity that can actually increase the likelihood of the best outcome under such circumstances.

We get to know our wounds and one another by being close and listening, not through battle. Like war between nations, it is impossible to know and understand the other side as long as one fights from a distance. Resistance creates resistance, force is met with force. We are part of nature that is so much bigger than any one of us alone. I know from my own experience that the patient works alongside the disease and with nature, surrendering deeper, dialoging, amplifying, and is initiated into new realms. Living in this way is associated with expansion, water, and renewal. One cannot resist a powerful wave but must flow with it.

Through my personal experiences with illness I learned that I can't hear the information illness brings if I treat it as a foreign invader. I have found a deeper connection to my body's natural reparative process by exploring illness through myths, stories, prayers, and dreams because it allows for a collaborative experience.

THE NURSE

Etymology of words is an intriguing way to reveal new insights. *Lymphaticus* in Latin refers to being seized by the nymphs. *Lympha* means nymph and water, and *lunaticus* is moon-sick or occasionally a bit crazy and a victim of the nymphs. Mythologically, cancer of the lymphatic system is about seeking water, being seized by the nymphs and moon-sick. Perhaps nymphs were unable to flow as the fluid in my lymph became diseased, a symptom of dryness without the moist feminine in my dry all-male, dusty, desert upbringing.

If we experience a traumatic event as if it is in some way divine, we find the capacity to survive beyond what we thought possible. A cancer diagnosis brings someone to a heightened awareness of what truly matters. The reality of illness linked to death reveals the divine. Illness may be an opening to a new relationship with the body's wisdom linked directly to the soul—a wake-up call that shakes one loose from a narrowly restricted life and releases one into the downward pull of instinct, desire, and joy.

Illness offers an opportunity for the soul to speak and convey what it desperately needs. Illness can open the patient to the necessity of the underworld journey when the psyche reveals secrets hidden in the body that may be toxic. Often something needs to die or be cut out so nature can do its job. The body works with nature in a reparative process. The nurse intuitively knows this.

In order to avoid the dangerous common trap of blaming patients for their illness, we must never forget that illness can also be just an illness of the body, and the body alone, with no larger meaning at all. It is always up to the patient to explore whether or not there is any sort of meaning.

The Nurse Today

The nurse works in a setting that is profane, yet her territory is sacred. When I first entered the profession, I heard the expression, "The nurse does what the physician and the janitor will not do." To this day I find this statement to be absolutely true. And it holds deep significance for the nurse because it is the nurse who takes care of the big messes and any confusing turmoil—emotional or physical—before the physician or the housekeeper will enter the room.

One of my former professors, Patricia Benner, often said, "There is an enormous difference between a novice nurse and an expert nurse." Today, experienced nurses are tired and overworked and often feel helpless in a system that does not fully support them. Nurses can be hard on new nurses and even belittle their naïvety. The new nurse is quickly disenfranchised by the red tape in healthcare. She hides her anger under a pleasing persona while depleting herself and may ultimately lose her center. The hardened veteran nurse sometimes withholds her expertise that is so desperately needed for the novice to begin her transformation. Nurses learn from nurses. A certain level of trust and openness is required in both directions. Otherwise, there is danger to patients inherent in lack of experience without good and consistent mentoring.

A nurse with experience not only has excellent clinical skills and intuition based on experience but also knows the importance of helping a patient maintain faith in what is possible. She helps patients sustain confidence in their capacity to get through a procedure, deal with a challenging diagnosis or event, and to face the future with new purpose. She knows there is an opportunity to guide the patient's experience by gently asking questions, listening carefully, and supporting individual, unique patients according to their needs.

The professional nurse is a negotiator, mediator, and diplomat. With the patient she downplays her knowledge and emphasizes her empathy which alleviates anxiety. The nurse asks questions to assess neurological status while simultaneously checking central lines, wounds, shifts in pattern, and facial expression. She gathers a myriad of data, unbeknownst to the patient, at every encounter.

There is a natural self-effacement in the nurse that I find absolutely endearing and delightful. She has been humbled over and over, well aware of the potential crisis around each corner. Mistakes will be made and, in spite of this, she is ready to respond with full attention, skill, and intellect at all times while juggling multiple tasks and interruptions. Any inflation of her ego is met with tenfold deflation. The ambiguity of the work requires humility.

Often nurses are told not to give information to a patient; then, when the physician does not share it either, it puts her in a difficult and all too common dilemma. Medical information withheld from a patient makes the nurse more uncomfortable than just about anything else. The nurse is a straight shooter who does not like to give false hope or engage in cover-ups.

Even though nurses in number make up the largest professional population in healthcare, they aren't covered in the news. Perhaps this is because they won't talk with media, especially about anything controversial. Hospital public relations departments insist that nurses conduct themselves outside work as a representative of the institution and remain silent about incidents, errors, or problems that may pose safety issues for patients and embarrassment to the institutions.

Nursing groups continue to try to get the media to improve the image of the nurse. The reason this hasn't worked is that we cannot simply change an archetype—it is too powerful and has staying power in the collective psyche. Media cannot change the image of the nurse because media is pulling from the same collective archetype and stereotypes as everyone else. Expanding each nurse's embodied experience of the nurse image is where it begins.

With more focus on technology, nurses still want to provide comfort and relieve suffering. Burnout comes when there is lack of true connection. Burn-out can feel like a death, and, in a way, it is. The soul hardens and there is a death of interest in the work. The calling withers. During these times of emptiness, the soul must at least go on wanting. As hopeless as it may feel, the character of the soul knows that the calling requires persistence. Paralysis and indifference impede all efforts to improve the situation.

Without claiming an authentic and effective voice, nurses often resort to abstract complaining and non-specific finger-pointing. They feel bad—hopeless and unappreciated—

but cannot articulate exactly why. With mandates from so many outside authorities who lack understanding of nursing practice, nurses go silent and refuse to do anything beyond their assigned duties. Rather than engage in a rebellious attempt to make positive changes in her working culture, the nurse is often complicit because she expects systems, like patients, to be unconscious, confused, and sick. Each nurse is individual in her impact, yet, without unity, nurses cannot be collectively proactive and major issues will not get resolved.

Currently, there are three million Registered Nurses in the United States. Nearly half are over 50 and only ten percent are under 30. Nurses are frustrated and tired in difficult working conditions, and there is a chronic shortage of nurses. Recent graduates are less satisfied and change jobs more frequently than others and 40% plan to leave within three years. Without young nurses, the profession is not being energized and renewed.

It cannot be overlooked that nursing is a dangerous profession. Safety is more and more an issue as the nurse takes on more complicated patients while supervising unlicensed personnel. The nurse responds to emergencies in awkward places such as small bathrooms or she tries to prevent a patient from falling, which leads to a back injury. Verbal and physical assault occurs as well as exposure to resistant bacteria, toxic chemicals, radiation, and a myriad of stressors. In the emergency room the danger is even greater, since many patients arrive intoxicated and trauma victims often have lethal weapons in their possession.

Sisterhood

The sisterhood of nursing is connected to womanhood, and nurses share a long ancestral bond based on conscious and unconscious memories and myths passed from generation to generation. The shared experience galvanizes this connection by nurses creating new stories and working closely together in a very intense environment.

Nursing as a sisterhood was promoted by Florence Nightingale. The shadow within the sisterhood today shows up as backbiting, fault-finding, and sabotage due to displaced anger and envy. Projecting and scape-goating within the sisterhood creates division, alienation, and furtherance of the status quo. Blaming others takes the place of personal responsibility and self-critique. A better strategy would be to create a safe environment where mistakes can be acknowledged, discussed, and explored. Every nurse remembers her first medication error. It is a rite of passage and the entire nursing staff shows love and empathy toward the new nurse when it happens. After that, there are incident reports and bad feelings, with little support.

Current nursing ethos does not promote shared myths and memories. Without rituals, ceremonies, and uniforms, there is a loss of identity. I lived in a dormitory for nursing students that was torn down in 2011. I ate all my meals at the hospital just across the courtyard. This isolation from the outside world was set up to foster learning, dedication, and characteristics of the ideal nurse. The stability, commitment, and endurance allowed nurses to flourish with the support of one another by living together throughout an intense initiation.

I grew up with all brothers. I find it easy to be the only woman in a large group of men. And, truth be told, men have never carried much mystery for me. At five years old, I began making friends with girls. I found them more interesting, challenging, and mysterious. I co-mingled with souls similar to my own. Never having had a sister and longing for nurturing feminine role models, I was called to the nursing profession. Nurses in some English speaking countries are still called "sisters." The sisterhood of nursing is a fundamental archetype. I found my home within nursing and have always loved it.

Before nursing was developed as a profession, rules about language, visitors, general behavior, use of alcohol and tobacco, sexual activity, and life in the hospital applied to nurses and servants who shared the same space and conditions as patients. Contemporary nurses often run errands and do secretarial and housekeeping duties as a matter of course. It is difficult for the nurse to delegate. A democratic approach seeking equality for all runs deep within the nurse.

Today's nurses collectively carry the origins of a profession that includes the poor, unskilled, criminals, and drunks and, at the opposite end, religious orders and the military. There is certainly evidence that characteristics from these foundations are active in today's nursing profession. In July 2009 the governor fired the top executives of the California Board of Registered Nursing because it was taking up to four years to get nurses with a criminal background into a database that could easily be accessed. Nurses who had been caught stealing drugs from work were allowed to continue to care for patients, and there was no system in place between law enforcement and the nursing board to be sure these nurses did not continue to work in other institutions until they had proved themselves responsible.

Mythologically, what does it mean to hide criminals within a profession? Is there a lineage that has not been fully acknowledged? Is this part of the shadow of compassion or forgiveness? Nurses react with action and fix things, yet it remains difficult to fire an incompetent or impaired nurse. There are re-trainings and diversion programs that are required before firing and a strong fear of litigation.

Nurses, who understand inequality in work life and understand interdependence with team members, have not strived for ultimate authority and power within the healthcare setting. During the women's movement, the nurse did not identify with the liberal feminist. She felt nurses would not likely gain equality, and feminism would alienate them from physicians. Now, nurses are more in line with the aims of feminism.

Although I would not know it for years, another reason I became a nurse was to take care of my father who had heart disease. As a new grad during a nursing shortage, I had the choice to work in just about any unit at Stanford. I chose oncology. I was unable to separate myself from the many patients who died of Hodgkin's Disease, the same disease I had had at age sixteen. I transferred to cardiology within the first year—an enjoyable position that also proved beneficial in keeping my father alive. I also went into nursing because I wanted to learn more about the feminine wisdom foreign to me since I grew up with men and a mother who colluded with them. I knew intuitively that there must be feminine wisdom in a career so dominated by women.

Nursing as a profession is in its infancy. Nurses are no longer who they were and do not know who they will become. The soul of the nurse is vast and receptive. There are endless possibilities for transformation. Nurses struggle to become more fully conscious, to speak out, and to develop an authentic voice. For the nurse it is about interdependent relationships while maintaining a genuine personal identity in collaboration with the soul of the nursing sisterhood.

CHAPTER 2
The Profession

In the 1850s, American hospitals were filthy, badly run, and populated mostly by the poor. Patients were often without beds, blankets, or pillows. People of means were cared for at home. There were few nurses at night except in cases of childbirth and impending death. Those in the role of nurse, mostly poor and untrained, worked without supervision and often drowned their grievances in alcohol, while others accepted bribes from patients.

Florence Nightingale (1820-1910) is the great visionary who established nursing as we know it today. She brought order to chaos and is mythic in her influence. She also contributed greatly in areas such as sanitation, clean water and air, nutrition, medical affairs, hospital construction, and statistics for public health, and penned signifiant works in spirituality and philosophy. Nightingale made altruistic patient care a covenant and used her intelligence, statistical knowledge, administrative skills, and political savvy to achieve her mission. Some of her philosophy seems restrictive by today's standards but those working as nurses then were in need of stringent rules and regulations.

THE SOUL OF THE NURSE

Nightingale, named Florence after the city in Italy where she was born, was from a wealthy family of Victorian England. She inherited what most would consider a life of luxury that included time for travel, study, and leisure. Yet she was often depressed. She questioned herself and was constantly in turmoil because she wondered why she got so little satisfaction from the privileged lifestyle many seemed to enjoy. It was a time when a woman was meant to be a wife and mother, with absolutely no outside interests. Women's duties included social engagements and spending most of their time in what Nightingale considered trivial domestic activities at home. Attending college and professional employment were not available to women. Since women could not earn a living, they married to survive. Those who were not wealthy worked in factories or as governesses and some supplemented their income with prostitution.

In 1852, Nightingale wrote "Cassandra," a crucial early feminist essay about the lack of opportunities for women. In it she makes known that women of her class are starving, desperate, diseased, and going mad due to their lives of inactivity and lack of engagement in their passions, intellect, and contribution to the world. With nothing of substance to do with their lives, she asserts, women don't even consider themselves human beings. In this essay, Nightingale laments that what she wants most is to attend a training program for nurses, but, since nursing is viewed as unladylike and beneath her class, she was forbidden to do so. She cannot fathom that society deems nursing so lowly a profession because, to Nightingale, nursing is the epitome of the love and care one human being can offer another. There is no higher goal.

In stating her personal philosophy, she asserts that she prefers suffering over indifference and pain over paralysis. She argues that nothing comes from nothing and out of suffering comes change. She says she'd rather die in the surf heralding the way than stand idly on the shore. She explains, "Passion, intellect, moral activity—these three have never been satisfied in woman. In this cold and oppressive conventional atmosphere, they cannot be satisfied. To say more on this subject would be to enter into the whole history of society, of the present state of civilization."

Nightingale railed against the plight of middle-class Victorian women. She demanded they be liberated from endless trivia to engage in a meaningful vocation. She felt that women accepted the world men created for them. She spelled out that girls are taught that "women have no passions" and "they *must* have none, they *must* act the farce of hypocrisy, the lie that they are without passion." Emphatically she adds, "Suffering, sad, female humanity! What are these feelings which they are taught to consider as disgraceful, to deny to themselves? What form do the Chinese feet assume when denied their proper development?"

She urges her reader to think about what makes a good female fiction character in novels. She says a woman is only interesting when she has high feelings and thoughts of character and no family ties—especially no mother—for that would interfere with her independence. She claims this is a perfect illustration of the damaging effects of family on women, holding them back from their true interests and career. The word *family* derives from Latin *famel*— servant, slave, a possession. *Father* derives from Latin *pater*—owner or master. So *pater familias* is the owner and master of slaves, his servants and possessions. And that was the world in which Nightingale lived. Fortunately, her father was more open to her intellectual and career aspirations. It was her mother and sister who attempted to confine her to a traditional role.

Nightingale reviled the common notion that women are meant to simply inspire and nurture men. She writes, "The family uses people, *not* for what they are, not for what they are intended to be, but for what it wants them for—for its own uses. . . This system dooms some minds to incurable infancy, others to silent misery." This condemnation of family sounds outrageously irreverent even today. Essentially, Nightingale brazenly asserted that family destroys individual life and creates women with no personal expectations. She declared that indeed many women want to be actively engaged in a career outside the home. She writes, "Marriage is the only chance (and it is but a chance) offered to women for escape from this death; and how eagerly and how ignorantly it is embraced!" And she concludes, "A man gains everything by marriage: he gains a 'helpmate,' but a woman does not." Her deepest conviction was that nursing is an inner calling based on intuition, and women have the right to make their own decisions, to marry or not, to work for something they believe in, and have a full and engaging career, all of which was unheard of in her day. Truly, Nightingale was defiant in the face of social mores. A true revolutionary.

The family tradition Nightingale found most deplorable was to be forced to listen to someone, usually her father, read out loud. She says children know this when they say, "Don't read it to me; tell it to me," which reveals her longing for myth through story telling and imagination. For Nightingale, being read the news or a book was, "Like lying on one's back, with one's hands tied and having liquid poured down one's throat." She craved interaction. She demanded intellectual give and take. In her late twenties she considered running away, dressing as a man, so she could attend college.

Nightingale craved time alone for contemplation and creativity which was severely denied. Her main gripe about being a woman in the Victorian Era was that women never were allowed time alone. The expectation was that women were responsible for entertaining others. Nightingale explains, "In social or domestic life one is bound, under pain of being thought sulky, to make a remark every two minutes." She felt under such circumstances nothing of substance was ever discussed because there was no time for contemplation or reflection. Nightingale's "Cassandra" influenced Virginia Woolf's revolutionary 1929 essay, *A Room of One's Own*, about the basic need women have for time alone to create. This theme was revisited in 1955 by Anne Morrow Lindberg in *Gift from the Sea*. Nightingale preceded Woolf and Lindberg in writing, "Time is the most valuable of all things." The theme of all three books is that women must make time to be alone in reflection with their inner life in order to find equilibrium in the complexity of life and the demands of being a woman.

THE PROFESSION

Nightingale engaged in an active dream life which was perceived in her day as narcissistic and trivial. She doubted herself and feared that her active fantasy and dream life was either a sin or a sign of mental illness. The world was to find out that suppressing a woman of Nightingale's enormous energy and capabilities leads to dramatic and revolutionary social change. She was a Mount Vesuvius ready to explode. Out of eruption came the birth of the nursing profession.

On the other hand, Nightingale was over-bearing, judgmental, and critical of women who did not have a work ethic, energy, and stamina to match her own. It disturbed her greatly when a colleague showed interest in personal life or marriage. She was all business yet, paradoxically, she wrote volumes on religion, mysticism, and spirituality. It was her stance that Jesus Christ raised women above the condition of slaves not to merely minister to the passions of men. She upheld that Christ's teachings liberated women to assume independent careers outside of raising children and it is up to humanity to give women the means to exercise these capacities. She wrote that nothing imaginable is more painful than the present position of women. Always a pragmatist, as mirrored by the profession she founded, she said, women must stop sitting and start doing something because, "Out of activity may come thought, out of mere aspiration can come nothing."

In her personal life, Nightingale fell in love and didn't marry. As always, she put her work first. She refused to put up with the repressive marital demands of the Victorian age. Victorian marriage did not foster partnership on any level. She hypothesized that if she and her partner could work together and combine their powers it would be a successful and happy marriage. The reality was that the husband had total control over his wife's money, assets, property, even her children and her body. Nightingale observed that marriage of her day did not feed the soul.

Nightingale's use of the Greek mythic figure, Cassandra, is no accident. She strongly identified with her. Nightingale's own prophecies, like Cassandra's, were often ignored. Akin to Cassandra, Nightingale understood the divine sounds of nature, specifically of birds. She even had a pet owl, rescued at the Parthenon. She named the baby owl Athena and carried it in her pocket. When the owl died it was stuffed and remains on display today at St. Thomas Hospital in London, site of her original nursing school.

Her essay, "Cassandra," expresses that a woman's voice is rejected and even mocked when she tells the truth. Nightingale embraced her mystical experiences as her most profound source of wisdom—such belief often deemed as hysterical. Society dictated that, the more a woman knows, the more she is neglected, hated, and ostracized. In "Cassandra," Nightingale succinctly enumerates the long-denied rights of women and reflects on the visions she had following travel in Egypt, Greece, and her secret visit to the German nursing school that laid the foundation for her career and purpose in life. She believed strongly the physical body is the holder of spirit made external through work in the world.

In the same year she wrote "Cassandra," Nightingale, at age 32, fulfilled her dream and began nursing training in Germany at a small hospital in Kaiserwerth where, for about a decade and a half prior to her entry, Pastor Theodor Fliedner and his wife Friederike had been training deaconesses. After her three month training, she accepted the position of superintendent of the Hospital for Invalid Gentlewomen in London where she immediately set forth to improve working conditions and concentrated on better ventilation and clean water. She believed that cramped spaces destroyed morale and increased drunkenness and crime within the hospital.

In 1854 the Nightingale legend was born when she organized a group of 38 women volunteers to nurse thousands of wounded and infected soldiers during the Crimean War. This is the Florence Nightingale commonly and nostalgically remembered by history.

To set the historical tone, in the nineteenth century physicians had little prestige and a very poor public image. Nightingale had an unfavorable opinion of them as well and envisioned a completely different role for nurses. She argued that medical training was not practical because it did not offer any cures. Treatments were limited to such things as purging, bleeding, and blistering. She felt the two professions ought to be kept distinct and women drawn to practice medicine should not see nursing as a short cut toward that goal. She felt men make fine nurses but, since she advocated for women and since men ran every other profession, she felt there was no need for them.

In order to keep lay-women from prescribing medicine, Nightingale set up the system we know today that requires medical orders to be written by physicians. Nurses do not prescribe but carry out doctors' orders. She set up the nursing hierarchy to be entirely administrated by nursing. Physicians take their concerns—hiring, disciplining, firing—to the nursing supervisor. This system is still in place today. She focused initially on recruiting farmers' daughters to be trained in her newly established nursing school, which is another compelling thread for me as my father was a rancher and farmer. She insisted that all classes of women should be allowed to enter the nursing ranks and that supervisors must go through the same training as any other nurse.

Nightingale did not believe all women make good nurses. She had strong opinions about who could qualify. After fourteen years developing the profession, she wrote a short primer, *Notes on Nursing*, to help women think like a nurse and bring general nursing concepts into the mainstream. Still, she strongly advocated that it was impossible to learn nursing from a book. She firmly believed that nursing was a hands-on experience that could only be truly mastered on the hospital wards.

Psychological by nature, Nightingale was quite aware of the subtle effects people have on one another. She therefore advised that a nurse work in a steady, calm, organized manner because the nurse's stress affected the patient. She made suggestions on how to interact with those who are ill. She said the nurse's touch must always be certain. She wrote, "Conciseness and decision in your movements, as well as your words, are necessary in the sick room, as necessary as absence of hurry and bustle."

She advised against visitors bringing "chattering hopes" to patients as it dismisses the gravity of their illness. She also said visitors should never bring any medical advice as the patient has likely heard it before and, if it worked, they would be doing it already. She said advice decreases the patient's confidence in their practitioners and the decisions they have already made about their care.

Nightingale shows herself to be a forerunner of depth and archetypal psychology in statements such as, "How often in such visits the sick person has to do the whole conversation, exerting his own imagination and memory, while you would take the visitor, absorbed in his own anxieties, making no effort of memory or imagination, for the sick person."

Her connection to nature was profound. She wrote that disease is "a reparative process. . . an effort of nature to remedy a process of poisoning or of decay." For Nightingale, it was nature, not medicine that would cure. She felt it is the nurse's job to put the patient in the best condition for nature to act. She insisted that cooperating with nature is the surest road to health.

On the practical side, Nightingale was a stickler for details. She was clear that observation and clear reporting are at the core of good nursing. She wrote, "If you cannot get the habit of observation one way or other, you had better give up the being a nurse, for it is not your calling, however kind and anxious [eager] you may be." Nightingale claimed the frustration nurses felt in communicating their opinions to physicians was based on their inability to communicate facts concisely and in as few words as possible.

Many authors suggest Nightingale feigned illness and was a wildly neurotic invalid. In fact, after she came down with brucellosis during the Crimean War, she was chronically ill with inflammatory pain, fevers, and bouts of fatigue for the rest of her very long life. Nevertheless, her illness did create the time so rare and so desperately needed for her contemplative and creative work. Illness, as she wrote, was the only excuse for a woman of her class to miss even one meal, social or domestic obligation. She writes, "Dinner is the great sacred ceremony of this day, the great sacrament. To be absent from dinner is equivalent to being ill. Nothing else will excuse us from it. Bodily incapacity is the only apology valid." Embracing her invalidism, she remained productive, writing and holding meetings in her home. She allowed only one visitor at a time, including her parents, in order to conserve energy. Unlike recluse American poet, Emily Dickinson of the same era, Nightingale made her presence known to all corners of the world through the ever-expanding British Empire. She was a force to be reckoned with, even from her sick bed. She died in 1910 at 90 of heart failure.

Not widely known, Nightingale was a prolific writer. According to Nightingale scholar, Barbara Dossey, her 14,000 letters have been available to scholars at the British Library and the Wellcome Medical Library for years. Her expansive genius has gone unrecognized until very recently. She had remained the stereotypical "lady with the lamp." Fortunately, her written works speak for themselves and many appear in the *Collected Works of Florence Nightingale* (16 volumes) that are astonishing in their breadth of practical, intellectual, and spiritual wisdom. Prior to this collection's publication, most of what was known about Nightingale was from limited secondary sources and she was widely misrepresented, so much so that the British nursing union in 1999, and the Royal College of Nursing in Edinburgh in 2000, removed Nightingale as the model for nursing. In 2001 the British Broadcasting Company portrayed Nightingale inaccurately as a right-wing conservative who opposed the women's vote and used religion as a front for her political activity. Nightingale was actually very liberal, with vast interests and always in favor of women's right to vote. She was debunked by this film when in reality the bulk of her political activity was focused on other women's issues specific to public health.

Florence Nightingale was imperfect. She was privileged, stubborn, a workaholic, and expected all nurses to give up their personal life. A product of the wealthy heavily patriarchal Victorian Era, she could be seen as out of touch with the reality of those with less talent and means. However, it is important that, when we look at figures who came before us, we do our best to look at them in historical context. She was allowed out of the family home only with her father's permission at the age of 32, and only after heart-wrenching personal perseverance. Nightingale is currently having a huge resurgence and is being embraced for her vast contribution and capacity for action.

Nursing in America

Before Nightingale's model of nursing made its way across the Atlantic, Dorothea Dix organized hospitals and nurses during the American Civil War. Simultaneously, Clara Barton brought the Red Cross to America. General consensus among Americans was that women, although mentally inferior to men, were morally and spiritually superior. In the United States nursing was seen as a disgrace to female modesty, piety, and delicacy. Consequently, there was a shortage of nurses and Walt Whitman (1819-1892) emerged as the voice of the nurse during the Civil War. His poem, "The Wound Dresser," draws sharp contrast between the sacred instinct of the nurse and the horror of war.

Attempts were made to train nurses in the United States after the Civil War, but the nursing field remained haphazard and disorganized. At New York's Bellevue Hospital, nurses were actually inmates released to undertake nursing duties in the wards as a type of punishment and form of community service. Each nurse was assigned at least twenty patients. The better hospitals were staffed by Catholic nuns and Protestant deaconesses, mostly untrained and with little knowledge of nursing.

In 1872, when socialites toured Bellevue Hospital, they found hundreds of dirty and distressed patients on the floor. It was generally believed that honorable women wouldn't be able to care for such patients. The statistics on morbidity and mortality were shocking, so the socialites decided to reform nursing training based on the Nightingale model. Nightingale schools paved the way for good training in the United States, although initially they lacked accreditation and had wide variations in curriculum until professional and legal regulations were implemented after the turn of the 20th century. Physicians objected to nurses who used medical terms or jargon or who showed they were learning from books, preferring that they carry out orders without question. This pattern of interpersonal relations extended to social life where interaction between the nursing and medical staff was strictly prohibited.

Socially, the nurse was aligned with the domestic, stenographer, and waitress—all occupations thought to threaten a woman's good character and behavior. The concern was that long hours of hard mental and physical work inclined nurses toward drugs and alcohol followed by sexual encounters with patients. In 1874, an essay in *Fraser's Magazine* about training schools for nurses claimed that nurses must learn to follow orders even if arbitrary and dictatorial—blind obedience and self abnegation were considered the foundation of good nursing. Student nurses were socialized to be submissive, hard-working, and loyal. Unpaid nursing students boarded in residence and made up a large portion of hospital nursing staff as they were called upon at all hours of day and night, often missing classes and losing sleep. The administrative argument was that it taught the perseverance and self-sacrifice necessary to be a good nurse.

THE SOUL OF THE NURSE

The nurse emerged as a professional due to the courage and ingenuity of Florence Nightingale and her volunteer nurses during the Crimean War. Future wars, each in its own way, heavily impacted the nursing field. Nurses surfaced as heroine figures after WWII in particular. Soldiers and the general public observed the nurse as cool under fire. She functioned admirably amidst the chaos and horrors of war. In the 1960s the nurse became the central most important factor, above the physician and technology, in the care of heart patients in newly opened Coronary Care Units. Nurse Practitioner programs also sprung up. Nurses championed health promotion and disease prevention during the era of feminism, environmentalism, and counterculture.

American advertisements featured the nurse image to promote a wide range of products including Wonder Bread, beer, appliances, airlines, and vibrators. The nurse was associated with healthfulness, cleanliness, efficiency, and safety. The negative emotion evoked by illness and hospitalization is balanced by the nurse's presence of comfort and hope for good health. This image continues to have commercial value today.

In the 1970s, with the shift toward a business model, hospitals observed that nurses were doing too many tasks below the level of their training and licensure, such as running specimens to the lab, stocking rooms, and giving baths. Cost savings were implemented by hiring less expensive staff. Reluctantly the nurse was forced to expand her role to include management and supervision, something in which she was not trained. Nurses began to work as a large collective and gain respect by working to change laws, and the role of Clinical Nurse Specialist emerged. By the 1980s the image of the nurse was positive, active, and benevolent, but not independent and powerful.

Nursing Now and in the Future

History sheds light on the nursing ideals of self-abnegation, obedience to authority, silence, doubt, and why the nurse hides her true power. For a century and a half, common obstacles have included inadequate staffing, constant interruptions, duplicative paperwork, cluttered noisy work stations, and lack of easy access to supplies. Yet the definitive issue remains that nurses have little decision-making power. They are employees of an increasingly business-oriented bottom-line industry. Today's nurse loves her work but hates her job.

The professional nurse deals with existential issues. She is on the front line for ethical dilemmas and is practical with cost-savings and waste reduction. She has proven to be a humanitarian and an economist. Nurses are the ones best suited to make final decisions about the services they provide.

Nightingale was openly defiant. She used the energy of her rage to move women into action and out of the status quo. There is an aching need for a shift that actually puts health first—health of patients, nurses, and other health professionals. Nightingale's ideas about the proximity to nature, clean air, window views, architecture, and quiet are now being considered and implemented. The nurse has historically instituted aesthetic modalities that have become mainstream like access to sun light, touch, music, flowers, and pet visitation, creating a warm ambience rather than cold sterility. It is time to go beyond these peripheral changes. Like Nightingale, it is time for the nurse to embody her central place in healthcare and focus on humanity to counter the current business and profit dominated system.

CHAPTER 3
Images of the Nurse

The topic of this chapter was so daunting that it took me a year to write. I resisted my personal visions and night time dreams. I was working in the traditional way—reading, doing scholarly research, and taking notes. Then, suddenly without warning, a chorus of wild and rapturous female voices implored me: "Please speak and tell the world who we really are!" The Dionysian maenads had arrived. They seized and liberated me, showing me how to break boundaries with this ambiguous material in an imaginal way.

Symbols of the Nurse

What came next surprised me. In search for the origins of the nurse, I was led to Marija Gimbutas who took me all the way back to prehistory. Gimbutas championed the controversial hypothesis that archaeological materials are not mute but actually speak a language of their own. This language allows present-day women to communicate with their foremothers. Gimbutas's all-important message for nurses is that the female of pre-historic times was not fragmented but whole. She once was indeed fully embodied in all her potential and power. Only after many millennia of willful male dominance did the female archetype become fractured. Today, the fully embodied female found in archaeological figures has all but been expunged. The nurse, like other females in mythology, has been systematically disassembled into smaller and smaller pieces and reduced even further in folklore.

Archetypal psychologist, James Hillman, added that the whole woman with her vast extremes is too terrifying for a male-dominated society to grasp, deal with, and understand. This is the reason she has been split and simplified. As a society we devalue feminine principles, as we do nature. Hospitals favor short-sighted quick fixes, spending on bricks and mortar rather than human-based care and programs for the ill. It's no wonder that women find it so difficult to fully engage their imagination. It is vitally important that we as nurses reawaken the whole woman inside each of us in order to reclaim our full capacity. Otherwise there is little hope for the current healthcare system.

Deprived of natural symbols nurses get stuck in ideologies. We look for ways to mourn the loss of our connection to natural rhythms. The nurse originates from the primal source— water. Expressions of the nurse from archeology are celebrated in the mysteries of the female body. We see in nature that animals lick the wounds of other animals and nurse other animals' offspring. When nature and the body are split, feminine power dissipates. When that split is translated into current hospital practice, the nurse and patients suffer because the full embodiment of the feminine has yet to be realized.

Prehistoric images associated with the nurse include the moon, springs, certain stones and animals. Each of these has its own expansive symbolism. The moon is associated with water, rain, and tides. It also brings floods and destruction. The moon rules the night where shadowy perceptions, instinct, and intuition prevail while the sun presides over the day and is governed by rational order. When the sun dominates, as it does in healthcare, the moon and stars are not visible. If the nurse is invisible, then elements of the instinctual and intuitive realm go unseen. Unfortunately, today's healthcare leaders are chosen for their solar qualities with little attention paid to their lunar sensibilities, creating an imbalance. Potential for transformation and renewal is lost.

Water

Prehistoric images of the nurse are connected to water, rain, and breast milk. Water is undefinable, shape-shifting, and able to conform to or break any container. Breasts, repositories of milk, are sacred because they hold the ever-flowing source of life. Flowing water purifies. Intravenous fluids are necessary for the hospitalized patient who is unable to eat or drink. Nurses have rituals around water including bathing, soaking, and washing hands. Now that most hospitals have mandatory hand-sanitizing dispensers I have concern for the drying effect on the nurse's hands and loss of hand washing as a ritual. Throughout the ages, water has been sacred and linked to improving strength, rejuvenating the weak, restoring sight, and purifying the body. Wells and thermal springs are connected to these powers. Life-giving female figures, like the nymphs, are commonly associated with wells.

Cup marks or hollows in stones symbolically represent miniature wells, the source of life-giving moisture. Those with disabilities seek relief by drinking this water, washing in it, or rubbing it on afflicted parts of the body. The nurse is habitually involved in multiple rituals involving containers and receptacles holding fluid. Today's nurse can give or withhold life-sustaining treatments including tube feedings and fluids. Symbols of the cosmic womb and vulva are found engraved on prehistoric rocks. Stones with holes are believed to be sacred with regenerative powers. Entrances to tombs with narrow vulva-shaped openings, like the one at Newgrange, County Meath, Ireland, allow the ritual of crawling through a narrow passage, symbolic of the birth canal, for regeneration simulating birth.

The belief in magical potency of streams and wells may explain why sanctuaries are often located near natural springs and mineral waters. Lourdes and Alsace of France, Esalen at Big Sur, and the natural springs of Germany are believed to have curative powers. Franklin D. Roosevelt, afflicted with polio, rejuvenated his spirit and resumed his political career that led him to the presidency, by bathing in natural hot-spring waters.

The constancy of the nurse can be likened to water carving out stone and moving past obstacles on its way to the sea. The drought, so common in many places and certainly part of my family mythology for five generations of ranching in central California, needs the moisture of female breasts, the flowing river of the vulva, the milk from cow udders, and the rain from the sky. Anyone who nurtures the world by bringing moisture, rain, or milk metaphorically is a nurse.

Animal Symbols

Gimbutas identifies the bird, snake, and bear as nurse symbols and the cow as the prehistoric animal symbol most commonly associated with the nurse. Udders and teats nourish. The shape of the cow's horns suggests the moon. I learned early in life on a cattle ranch what my father meant when he said I needed to separate "wet" and "dry" cows. No explanation was given. I figured out that the large swollen udders meant wet cow and shriveled up udders meant dry cow. The dry cows were sold because they would not produce a calf that year. My father attempted to protect me from the harsh reality of ranch life. We never discussed that I was helping decide the fate of each cow and in all likelihood sending the non-productive cows to their deaths.

Like the nurse, cows have natural tendencies toward being gentle, trustworthy, docile, and compliant with domestication. The cow as metaphor balances docility and strength. There is humility in recognizing limitations. Cows are also tough and can be fierce under certain circumstances. The downside, when the tough and fierce aspects of the nurse are forced underground, as in the current medical hierarchy, is that the nurse learns ways to manipulate others to get what she needs. One tactic is to exaggerate her helplessness to avoid confrontation.

Today's nurse is often stereotyped as an angel of mercy wearing a cap and uniform. Archeological findings predate this image as the woman with wings. The bird woman sometimes has snakes on top of her head and she is often seated on a royal throne. This suggests the possibility that the nursing cap has a powerful, even regal, significance. The bird and snake goddess hold transformative powers around life and death. She protects, nourishes, and regenerates. She goes beyond other archeological figures that represent fertility and motherhood. The nurse in this way is specifically remembered in prehistoric artifacts.

Also associated with the nurse are water birds. When my mother was dying I observed more geese and herons on the creek that runs through the ranch. One of the few times my mother and I were alone, a snake appeared coiled on the floor between her hospital bed and the sofa where I slept. My fear of the snake was unwarranted as I could see it was not poisonous or a rattlesnake. My destructive impulse took over. I grabbed a broom and swept the snake outside through the sliding glass doors where it was taunted by a cat. My mother died the next day, less than six months after my father. Only later did I grasp the connection between the snake as symbol of protection and regeneration and the mother-daughter immortality mystery. In almost every culture snakes symbolize renewal. They hibernate, awaken in spring, transcend boundaries from the depths of the earth, and slough their skin. They are representatives of the underworld and the ever changing continuity of life. The royal snake, like her bird sister, guards life-water and life-milk.

The bee, butterfly, and owl are also associated with the nurse. Bees not only provide nourishing honey but are necessary to the ecosystem, just as the nurse is necessary to the functioning of the healthcare system. Butterflies emerge from a worm-like state in a cocoon and, like the snake, symbolize regeneration. On the other hand, owls mean something different to different cultures. There is no one set of consistent beliefs, other than that owls are revered and generate fascination and awe. Native Americans on both continents regard the owl as the harbinger of death. Some mythologies see owls as bad omens, while many hold the owl in high esteem. Florence Nightingale valued the owl as her favorite bird. The owl, like the nurse, is both feared and venerated, associated with witchcraft, sorcery, wisdom, the night, and death. The patient comes to the hospital in a vulnerable state, relying on treatment and care by the nurse in order to either emerge newly regenerated like a butterfly or complete their life cycle through death, aided and symbolized by the owl.

IMAGES OF THE NURSE

The night before my father died I was driving on a dark dirt road back to the ranch after sitting with him at the hospital. An owl suddenly appeared in front of me. I was forced to stop the car. Even when I started to roll forward, the owl would not move. I sat eye to eye with the owl for several minutes and considered the depth and intimacy of the moment. I knew I needed to be back with my father early the next morning for what proved to be his final breath. It was as if the owl waited until I got the connection before its huge wings opened and it flew off into the moon light.

In fairy tales the death-wielding and destructive aspect of the female has been degraded to a witch or crooked old woman with a large pointed nose like the bird of prey. The death messenger appears as a slim, ugly woman dressed in white or might be heard as a bird squawking or flapping its wings near the house when a person is about to die. Nurses have worn the color white up until recently and many still wear white lab coats. The color is thought to be pure—perhaps a desexualization. However, the prehistoric meaning of white is associated with death, the color of bone. Red, the color of blood, is associated with life.

The nurse is also linked to the toad. Nocturnal and mysterious, the toad is associated with the womb. Since the cause of conception was not fully understood, it was concluded that a toad crawled into the womb and became an embryo. This was likely surmised because a miscarried human embryo at one or two months looks very much like a toad. I collected toy toads and frogs as a pre-teen. Perhaps my unconscious was already drawing me to the nocturnal, instinctual, and mysterious.

The bear, in mythology, is connected to initiation and rites of passage, protecting the initiate while vulnerable. The bear also represents the fierce and destructive aspect of the nurse; like the fully embodied female of prehistory, she not only creates but destroys. Initiation is a ritualistic experience of rebirth. It involves entry into the depths of the underworld and re-membering what has been forgotten. Symbolically this destruction is necessary to make way for new life and, often, a new role in the world. Nurses wearing animal masks and pouches on their backs are common prehistoric symbols. The hump on the back signifies a pack containing supplies. Today's nurse with poor posture and sore back resembles the prehistoric bear nurse who is carrying a heavy load on her shoulders. Split off from her own body and emotions, she bears the weight of others on her painful and numbed body. The bear can be gruff, burly, and bad-mannered.

IMAGES OF THE NURSE

Fairy Tales

Fairy tales are more than simple stories for children. They stimulate imagination, entertain, and help sort out inner turmoil. A rich fantasy life mixed with reality is necessary for personal development. The truth of fairy tales exists only in the imagination. This is why fairy tales do not need to be moral. Morality implies conformity to right and wrong which prevents access to paradoxical feelings, urges, and passions. Fairy tales are a safe fantasy outlet for darker perceptions. The monster can be useful if it allows us to work through feelings of helplessness and anxiety. Like communication with an illness, these stories expand our options, make us more flexible and open to unforeseen outcomes. If there is a bad witch, in a tale she can be crushed by a house or put in an oven and burned up. Once we become familiar with her, her fearsome aspects fade and reassuring aspects begin to surface. This is similar to why we seek the thrill of roller coasters and why we feel so good when we make it through the ride. Medications such as tranquilizers blunt the evolution of anxiety. They don't allow us to face it, master it, and be transformed by it.

Fairy tales present brief dilemmas with very little detail and simple characters. They foster hope by allowing success through trickery. They show that even the meekest can succeed. Fairy tales tend to be about feeling significant and loved. They present our fear of annihilation. In fairy tales it is easy to see good versus evil, stupid versus clever, and industrious versus lazy. In contrast, myths are more complex. Fairy tales are presented as if they could happen in everyday life while myths play on larger themes. Mythic figures often seek immortality, destiny, and legacy while the fairy tale protagonist seeks merely to live happily ever after on earth. Happily ever after means forming a satisfying bond to someone else in order to dispel the fear of death. By demonstrating how to form true interpersonal relationships, fairy tales teach us how to let go of parents and personal ancestry. They lessen our fear of growing old.

Fairy tales expand the imagination beyond narrow confines and preoccupations. This is important for the nurse, especially as she ages. When we are young we have uncompromising idealism and moral rigidity and believe anything is possible. In midlife we move toward a more tragic insight. We accept that we cannot control things and that people have various ethical principles and differing perspectives. Through experience we learn to tolerate limitations and accept that there is evil in the world. The soul longs to expand its repertoire. If people do not cultivate imagination and creativity, they simply grow old and become increasingly resentful and angry. Fairy tales offer innovation and insight. The tendency is for the nurse to get stuck, as healthcare is stuck, in old stories that lack inventive solutions and fresh approaches. In addition to stimulating the imagination, fairy tales stir up eros and passion. Like her primal symbol, water, the nurse needs to flow. Fairy tales keep us from getting stagnant.

How the Nurse Appears in Fairy Tales

The nurse appears frequently in fairy tales. She nourishes men and ministers to children, often tending to those who have been abandoned. Nurses sometimes use trickery for escape and even kill and cook children and feed them to their parents. Nurses show powers of perception and recognition, sometimes they are clever, other times they are short-sighted with absurd plans. Nurses are thieves, tricksters, sometimes fatally deceptive, and are depicted as adulterers, and impostors. Nurses have a nose for hypocrisy. They are not above begging alms to nurture a child, exchanging children for financial gain, or playing favorites by helping a select few gain wealth. The nurse rescues, revealing herself as a divine helper and occasionally as a demigod. She is often used as a disguise. She evokes surprise, admiration, and wonder. In the *Stith Thompson Motif Index of*

THE SOUL OF THE NURSE

Folk Literature the nurse shows up most commonly under the following categories: animal helper, deception, the wise and the foolish, and marvels. These themes play out in art and other narratives as well.

Nurses in Mythology

Before classical myths were written down, people lived close to nature. They were in tune with seasonal changes and the natural rhythms of the female body. The Olympians of Greek mythology split the female—Hera as jealous wife of Zeus, Hestia as invisible keeper of the home, Athena as cold warrior, Aphrodite as sexual object, and Artemis as the forgettable sister of Apollo. There are many familiar, mostly reductive, personality characteristics of the nurse seen repeatedly in mythology that represent her many guises. Psychologically, gods and goddesses of mythology represent specific patterns of behavior that reside in the collective. When we suppress our most authentic and natural behavior symbolized by one of these gods or goddesses, we metaphorically dishonor them, and ourselves. When we anger them, they make themselves known in unexpected ways. For instance, whenever I attempt a lifestyle that has a rigid schedule, Dionysus is sure to sabotage my efforts with good food, wine, and friends who like to revel late into the night.

The following nurse figures are presented in the order in which the myths appeared. Longer sections are devoted to the more complex and specifically relevant nurse mythological figures.

Ninshubur: Nurse as Faithful Servant

Inanna is considered one of the first Western myths. In it, Inanna, Sumerian queen of heaven and earth, descends into the underworld to face her sister Ereshkigal. Inanna implicitly trusts her nurse, Ninshubur, to keep her safe as she moves deeper and deeper into increasingly dangerous territory. Ninshubur as her advocate is responsible for her rescue. She enlists Enki, god of waters and wisdom, to help her. Enki creates tiny rescuers that are able to slip into the underworld with food and water. The tiny rescuers show compassion and acknowledge the suffering of Ereshkigal. Touched by their empathy, Ereshkigal allows them to take Inanna's corpse, which they revive and return to the living.

Inanna then must find a replacement for herself in the underworld. She decides Dumuzi, her husband, rather than Ninshubur, will take her place. And there is an important reason for this. Ninshubur never left her when she was vulnerable, while Dumuzi enjoyed his reign far too much in her absence. Inanna's rebirth serves as a powerful metaphor for initiation into healthy womanhood. Ninshubur is deeply reflective and functions best when Inanna is most threatened. Her capacity for action at the precise moment is extraordinary yet she remains nearly invisible and behind the scenes with integrity and reverence.

Nut: Nurse as Life Cycle

As the great mother figure of Egyptian mythology, Nut arches over the earth, protecting humanity with her body. She nurtures with her breasts and milk. She is associated with the cow. Nut, mother of the dark night sky, allows stars and planets to shine. She devours the sun, Ra, in the evening and rebirths him at dawn. Nut was dismissed to the sky because she was eating her young. Her devouring aspect and ability to regenerate is symbolic of the natural life cycle the nurse is so familiar with. Nut is represented on the lid of coffins and sarcophagi. Perhaps symbolically today, nurses are missing the affirmation piece by eating young novice nurses and forgetting the regeneration piece necessary to the health and survival of the profession. Nut gave birth to four children, Osiris, Isis, Seth, and Nephthys.

IMAGES OF THE NURSE

Isis/Hathor: Nurse as Re-memberer

Isis, later Isis/Hathor, is very close to the nurse mythologically. She puts Osiris back together again after he is murdered by Seth who usurps his throne. Isis recovers Osiris's casket and puts it in a barge. When Seth returns in a rage, he dismembers Osiris and scatters him. Isis then navigates treacherous seas by boat, collects the scattered pieces, and puts Osiris back together again. She cannot find his penis, so she constructs one and hovers over his body like a kite-bird and is impregnated. The product of their union is Horus. Ancient statues of Isis nursing Horus were renamed by early Christians as the Virgin Mary and Jesus.

Isis uses deception, trickery, and magic to help Horus achieve the throne. Horus then beheads her after she shows compassion for Seth. She is given a cow's head and restored to life. From then on she is known as the Horned Crescent, Hathor. Despite all her dismemberment, Isis/Hathor perseveres. Images show her cow head adorned with a throne, sun disc, and horns. Sometimes she has wings. She guides, protects, and helps those in need to overcome obstacles. She is called upon in times of injury and knows how to heal common ailments, like rashes, sprained ankles, and flu, through use of her voice, bread, beer, wine, herbs and her body fluids.

THE SOUL OF THE NURSE

She protects women and represents pleasure, music, and dancing. Her exuberant parties and orgies predate the drunken orgiastic revelry of the Dionysian maenads. Isis/Hathor when angry manifests as Sekhmet, a raging destructive lioness who inflicts diseases and also knows how to remedy them. Isis/Hathor displays the full range of the fully embodied female. She has the capacity to both nurture and destroy.

Greek Nurse Mythological Figures

Greek mythological figures that display some characteristics of the nurse include Artemis, Athena, Aphrodite, and Pandora. What follows is a snap shot of each.

Artemis protects women during childbirth. She is the virgin huntress who reveres wild life. The bear is sacred to her and nine year old girls are her playmates. Tithenidia is the festival of nurses in Sparta held in her name. She is Apollo's twin and associated with the moon.

Athena stands on guard protecting her territory as the nurse does her patients. She is astute at noticing every person and she is suspicious if people look like they do not belong. Associated with the owl, she wears a shield and is ready to attack any enemy that encroaches. Nurses, especially in critical care, personify the energy of Athena.

Aphrodite, born of the sea, is aquatic and associated with the water bird. The shell is her sacred symbol. She embodies sexuality. She is the inspiration behind the ancient legend of the holy prostitute who reintegrates soldiers into civilized society after the savagery of war. Modern nurses have been either desexualized in their white starched uniforms or perverted into pornographic figures. Aphrodite defends physical love and fleshly union and also finds expression in manipulation and coyness.

Pandora is the Greek Eve, the first woman of ancient patriarchal Greek mythology. She is best known for unleashing evil into the world. The myth shows that she promises beauty, pleasure, and power yet turns out to be an empty and destructive temptress with insatiable desires. Pandora is alive and well in our materialistic culture where females learn how to present themselves as objects of desire to attract and control men. Ultimately seduction and false beauty sacrifice women to the collective ideal.

Hygeia: The Silent Nurse

For most, the Greek mythological nurse figure that first comes to mind is Hygeia, goddess of health. She is the daughter of Asclepius, the god of healing. Her actual role is unknown and there are no stories about her. Perhaps Hygeia holding the snake close to her body symbolizes regenerative health while her sister Panacea is the restorer of health. Mistletoe, which hangs from oak trees and looks like genitals thus symbolizes procreation, is associated with love and kissing during the holidays and is linked to Hygeia. Hygeia is a prominent figure frequently seen yet always silent at the side of Asclepius. This image has had a lasting impact on the nurse-physician relationship. Hygeia is mute. She does not speak or have a voice of her own. She remains very distant, perhaps as helpmate, yet never in full partnership with the physician.

Baubo: Bawdy Body of Revelry

In contrast to Hygeia, Baubo is shamelessly outspoken and in my opinion the most delightful nurse in Greek mythology. She embodies the personality of today's nurse. She brings the naked truth to light through wit, impropriety, and her bawdy body humor. She serves as nurse to the harvest goddess, Demeter, who is beset with rage and sorrow over losing her daughter, Persephone. Baubo lifts her skirt exposing her vulva which shocks Demeter and makes her laugh. This life-affirming gesture is linked to Aphrodite and suggests that grief, mourning, and self-regulation need to be countered by wild instinctual sexuality to restore equilibrium. Baubo remains Demeter's most trusted nurse and companion.

Baubo also consoles Demeter with barley-water that may have hallucinogenic properties. She sings salacious songs to relieve emotional tension. Her profanity brings Demeter down to earth. Baubo belongs more to women than men and has no interest in the rules of patriarchy. She shakes with belly laughter. She dances for Eros and Aphrodite bridging the gap between the raunchy, muddy instinctual nature and the transcendent realm. She reminds us that women can experience so much pleasure in their bodies.

Sometimes Baubo images show her as a gorgon with skeletal ribs and head, maintaining large genitalia––death and regeneration inseparably linked. Baubo-like images and figures existed in Paleolithic, Neolithic, Hellenistic, Egyptian, and medieval times. The skirt-raising gesture, *ana-suromai*, was also demonstrated by Hathor in Egypt. Women's rituals, as far back as prehistoric times, were rowdy celebrations with music, humorously indecent merrymaking, offerings, wine, clowning, joking, and exposure of breasts and genitalia from boats and from shorelines of rivers.

Baubo, like the nurse, often plays the important role of old fool. Our culture expects everyone to become a wise elder thus diminishing the importance of the old fool. Old fools express likes and dislikes bluntly, are not driven by money, and know they do not have ultimate power. They have freedom to be creative, enjoy life, say what they want, and behave as they wish. Old fools laugh and cry and speak the truth unrestrained like children. Old fools in mythology and folklore make everyone feel good because they don't intimidate anyone.

Hermes: Nurse as Psychopomp

Hermes is the great communicator and messenger. His mother was a nymph or nurse. Like Baubo, he does not demand formality or good manners. He breaks taboos and blurs lines. He lives on the margins and is familiar with unchartered territory. He is able to move in and out of situations easily. Both Baubo and Hermes use jokes and trickery to achieve desired ends and delight in eroticism, humor, and pranks without doing harm or being destructive.

Hermes protects travelers. His pace is always rapid as indicated by the wings on his hat or feet. He appears suddenly as a divine messenger. C.G. Jung calls the figure who mediates between the conscious and unconscious worlds a psychopomp. As psychopomp, Hermes is the god people pray to when dying, the trusted escort who knows the way to the underworld. He takes souls to their death and can bring them back from the dead. Nocturnal, he is also the guide of dreams. Uncertainties and dangers are calmed by his kind presence.

Hermes, sometimes seen with Hygeia, has practical wisdom and is skilled with fire, splitting wood, roasting meat, and pouring wine. Hermes guards with craftiness, deception, and luck. He loves unscrupulous profit and the ways of women. He is lucky in love and is able to increase herds. Hermes, as nurse, is not heroic but a practical indispensable servant.

Hecate: Intensity at the Crossroads

Hecate holds more nurse traits than any other mythic figure. Like her companion, Hermes, Hecate is a psychopomp, always in the shadows, a guide for other souls. She moves easily between clarity and disorientation, truth and deception, and teaches how to live on the edge. Hecate is perceptive and able to hear what others cannot. She has no relatives and has learned from her own abandonment how to be with others in their suffering. Guardian to nurses, she bears witness to people in crisis, the situation where she is most comfortable. In contrast to Apollo, she's at home with wild emotions. This is the realm of the nurse— constantly seeking intensity. Associated with nightmares and the rhythms of the female, Hecate does her work in darkness. She has a strong masculine side that supports her feminine sensibilities.

The Erinyes are nurse companions to Hecate. Connected to the deep earth, they demand justice and answers. Sometimes winged like angels, Erinyes resemble the predatory Harpies, with a voice of lowing cattle or Hecate's barking dogs. Like Florence Nightingale, Hecate carries a torch, symbolizing the light of understanding and intelligence. The torch, like the moon, can rekindle a broken heart. Hecate's secret kind of lunar knowledge is not Apollonian—not a rational kind of thinking. She is intuitive and clairvoyant. She embodies crossings, departures, beginnings, and endings. Hecate is protector of Hecuba who is thought to be a witch and is mother of Cassandra.

Cassandra: Nurse as Medium

Cassandra does not need approval nor does she attempt to meet the desires of others. She belongs to herself alone. She is a medium who foretells many disastrous prophecies. She is able to see what is hidden. Although her predictions are absolutely correct, she is disregarded and ultimately martyred for speaking up. She is truly a tragic figure because she possesses wisdom and insight yet is powerless to convey it.

IMAGES OF THE NURSE

Nurses, like Cassandra, are intuitive and often see things before others do. All nurses have been scolded for speaking up and "over-stepping" their boundaries. The Cassandra tale illustrates the disastrous consequences that can ensue when a nurse's insight is dismissed. Dominating masculine values often leave the nurse's voice marginalized and unexpressed. The nurse who cannot speak up represses her skill, experience, and knowledge which leads to rage and agitation. She swallows so much injustice that she feels helpless and is in conflict with her inner authority.

Dionysian Maenad: Nurse as Ecstatic Nymph

Sex, death, and the underworld belong together mythologically and find full expression through Dionysus. He is irresistible and does not exploit females. Without a mother, he was raised by nymphs, or nurses, later called maenads. A nymph is a goddess or a mortal unwed maiden who inhabits springs, wells, and marshy lowlands. Like the nurse, the element of water is her origin. Dionysus naturally loves nurses and everything about women. He sweeps women off spiritually from their daily work, liberating them into instinctual womanhood.

Women in touch with this power know that dance, song, and sexuality are as necessary for survival as food preparation and raising children. A nurse allowing herself to act according to instinct, without conscious criticism of what she does, and without paying attention to the implication of her words and deeds, threatens conventional values and standards. Although these standards have been established to curtail unconscious instincts, every woman knows she has them. When rules become sterile and predictable, women yearn even more for a way to contact the source which springs from her unimpeded urges.

Today the Dionysian spirit is on display at funerals that turn into drinking festivals. Dionysus links death with life's exuberance. Getting drunk and being sexually audacious and playful are ways of asserting life in the face of the harshness of death. Nurses face grim situations every day and are known for their wild parties and gallows humor. Since nurses work so closely with death, it is natural that they become possessed with the wanton spirit of Dionysus.

Maenads live out-loud; nothing is held back. They are comfortable in their body, absolutely unbridled and unrestrained. Maenads express wild ecstatic love and full-blown rage. Our culture has no ritual outlet for this type of release, so we numb our impulses. Dionysus brings on mania, eroticism, animal consciousness, and revelations. He is patron of theater and histrionics. The nurse merges with Dionysus in the drama and mayhem of her daily work. She often has sudden insights yet feels a bit less than sane when she attempts to voice her epiphanies.

Dionysian exuberance and euphoria, are rooted in life's inevitable wanting, hunger, thirst, vacancy, and waning hope—all vital for a healthy emotional life. The nurse chronically faces immensely difficult situations involving heroic treatments with patients on the border of life and death. The nurse wants and needs a way to affirm life, especially in times of decreasing hope. Longing is healthy yet the expression of wanton behavior is linked to immoral and lewd acts, implying poor breeding and education. Displaying uninhibited, undisciplined lust, like the Dionysian maenads, is censured and condemned.

Vigilance is an absolute necessity in critical and acute care where the nurse provides highly skilled expertise. Often the nurse faces contradictory wishes from loved ones and healthcare team members. Where is the outlet for the nurse? Where does she loosen her instincts? How can her thirst be quenched? Thirst, from earliest symbolism, is the central craving of the nurse. Dionysus calls nurses instinctually to wild frenzy and intoxication to affirm life and burn away their harsh reality.

Without replenishment how can the nurse live an intensely emotional and spiritually charged life?

Some religious sects use intoxicants and hallucinogens to transcend the mundane. Mind altering substances serve two purposes, the worshipper is able to gain release from everyday life and connect with the divine. In our pent-up world, it is the letting go that is missing. How and where does the nurse take this symbolic and necessary leap? How does she surrender, loosen, let go, and give over conscious control? Where does she go to allow inspirational impulses to flow? The modern healthcare system is split off from the Dionysian. The nurse serves the Apollonian, which is a more distant mechanical experience of medicine. Unlike Hygeia, today's nurse is not meant to simply remain silent and support the masculine. Merging with Dionysus releases the nurse's true feminine potential.

Dionysus and Apollo

Dionysus and Apollo are diametrically opposed. Dionysus rides on the full fury of life force as the great loosener and stirs things up when they get too rigid. Apollo focuses on differences of form and maintains order at all cost. Apollo, exacting and hierarchical, represents an unreachable perfectionism. Apollo remains distant in order to see form clearly, whereas Dionysus must touch to merge with soul. Nursing, although different at its roots and origin, has followed the Apollonian medical model, forgetting Dionysus. Nurses are not machines, nor are their patients. As James Hillman writes, "The force of life needs nursing. The Dionysian experience transforms women not into raving hysterics and rebels but into nurses."

The nurse, like the ancient Egyptian Ra, is consumed in death and regeneration daily. Mania is her birthright. The rigid Apollonian mindset cannot exist without the freeing aspect of the Dionysian. Mania is actually necessary and a sort of divine madness. In this state there is an urgent desire to produce something real and genuinely alive. It begins with the impulse to create without normal controls in place. In fact it means turning them off. Possession by the Dionysian maenads requires diving to the very depths where eros and death live.

The women of the water who surround Dionysus are his beloved nurses. The archetypal feminine world, at its core, conforms to nature—not morals, rules, laws, or marital or domestic duties. Maenads show the paradox of nature through their nurturing and protective side as well as in their mad and destructive side. The two basic drives of love and death— relatedness and oblivion—show up symbolically in the maenads' euphoric exaltation and blameless destructiveness.

Because Dionysus is tethered in the liminal space between life and death, he suffers. He is connected to the depths of the underworld and, whenever the underworld is agitated, there is rapture, birth, horror, and destruction. What is below generates what comes to the surface. New life always comes out of the abyss. The nurse as maenad also suffers. Continual creation requires generation and destruction. Sending a bird out of the nest, or a child out of the house when time, is like killing, so devouring is also a way of being protective. Dionysus symbolizes the torture of not being remembered and calls the soul to vulnerability—to where it is wounded most.

Dionysus is also the tender lover, the nurturer, the bearer of wine that removes anxiety and worry. He also eats raw flesh and symbolizes human sacrifice. Some suggest meat dripping with blood represents the vitality and sexual potency of Dionysus. He is sometimes torn limb from limb; other times he dismembers others—his life a constant cycle of being devoured and absorbed. Wherever ambivalent feelings appear there is an opening for Dionysus. Compulsion and inhibition are aligned in Dionysian consciousness.

IMAGES OF THE NURSE

Dionysian victories come from wine and indirect, subtle, clever, sometimes perverse, manipulation of enemies. Breaking out of bondage of law, duty, and custom requires Dionysian madness. Oppression of passion and the creative impulse in today's nurse creates agitation. She is repressed and dissociated. Distortions arise from this turmoil and we witness the return of Dionysus who insists on being present. Dionysian strength and power by definition is feminine. Apollo portrays it as weakness and passivity. Its characteristics are dark and obscure, leaning toward melancholy.

Nurses have objectified both their work and home life in an Apollonian way. Like Athena, the nurse is a true warrior, protecting her people, yet she has no armor. With pain killers, sleeping pills, drinking too much alcohol, she attempts to soothe the soul that is so neglected. Nurses use "spirits" in a literal attempt to connect with spirit. Today's rituals do not educate her and reinforce the paradoxical nature of her work. She acts out through obsessive-compulsive behavior, outbursts, passive-aggressiveness, and manipulation. Her body calls out in physical sensations and ailments attempting to say, "I desire. I long for the depths. I want to be alive in the vast ocean of the unconscious, embracing vulnerabilities, loving and being loved." She needs to connect with her divine creative energy. Yet there is no safe place to express her raging anger, her exuberant passions, and let herself go completely.

Adaptation to convention simply weakens us. Distractions feel cheap and fleeting. Once the soul decides to descend, there is no way to deter it. Breaking out of bondage threatens those around her. Yet, she must leave her neatly packaged life. She is seized by the Dionysian maenads at places she most carefully guards. Initiation into womanhood is primal, an ancient ritual displayed in the frescoes of Pompeii. Dionysus shakes the nurse loose from her narrow restricted life and pulls her down into animal instincts and desires which she cannot resist.

The nurse, raised to have good-girl standards, will be appalled, outraged, and distressed at those very places she has maintained as acceptable and proper. Her very foundation will crumble. Dionysus offers emancipation from Apollonian domination. He responds to necessity. Where order reigns, he is in frenzy. Where the sexes are too rigidly defined, he is bisexual. Where there is fragmentation and isolation, he generates community. Where is there more attempted order, control, and sterility than in a hospital?

IMAGES OF THE NURSE

Today's nurse is dissatisfied. There are no living images that reflect her vast complexity and wholeness. Neolithic symbols, folklore motifs, and mythology connect the nurse to the regenerative cycle. Imagine a ritual today in which the new initiate returns from the depths of her experience, all alone, to waiting sisters that know and understand where she has been and help her regain her wits and power of laughter. This community exists now if we make it part of our contemporary rite of passage.

CHAPTER 4
The Nurse in Popular Culture

Film captures the spirit of our age and is an obvious place to find the nurse in popular culture. Nietzsche proclaimed, "We have art so that we shall not die of reality." Nurses in film and television, however, are mostly secondary characters. Most show the nurse as marginalized in some way, with little professional autonomy, doing insignificant tasks. Often physicians are shown performing nursing functions like starting an IV. The films I've chosen reflect the most common traits of the nurse and convincing characters. I've also included some images from literature and art. Rather than reject any of these portrayals, my approach has been to explore these characters, no matter how farfetched and unbearable. The eleven following categories emerged organically.

Power-Hungry Villain

Hostility toward nurses shows up in art, literature, and film, almost as if it belongs there. As the step-mother is in fairy tales, the nurse is manipulative, controlling, and dangerous. Characterized as unresponsive or over-bearing, the nurse is the insider, the guide in the uncertain domain of illness, wrought with powerful emotions. Two unforgettable films, *One Flew over the Cuckoos Nest* and *Misery*, portray extreme examples of the unyielding, sadistic, malevolent nurse.

The Academy Award-winning role of Nurse Ratched, played by Louise Fletcher, in *One Flew over the Cuckoo's Nest* (1975), adapted from Ken Kesey's novel, brings to life the best known one-dimensional nurse in film. When I tell people I am writing about the nurse, almost in unison they cry out, "Do you mean Nurse Ratched?" Even Fletcher said in her acceptance speech, "It looks like you all hated me so much that you've given me this award. . . All I can say is I've loved being hated by you." The audience laughed knowingly because we all love and hate the nurse. Although Ratched is an all-powerful matriarchal figure, the film is set in a patriarchal mental institution and beset with sterility. Rather than displaying the brutal dehumanization set up by the male-dominated mental health system, Ratched, herself, is in control.

She wears the traditional starched white uniform and cap. Out from bloodless white skin stare steely-blue eyes. She has a monotone voice and is never ruffled. Her controlled demeanor is in itself terrifying. She claims that loud classical music benefits patients when actually it drowns out their baseball game on television. Ratched threatens rectal suppositories to anyone refusing medications. She has no sense of humor and no tolerance for gambling, sex, and anything that feels out of her control. She is oppressive and suffocating in her role.

The tension of the film revolves around the free-spirited newcomer McMurphy, played by Jack Nicholson, who also won the Academy Award for his role. Ratched provokes her patients' outbursts and vicariously lives through them, commenting that there is freedom in being committed because you are allowed to act crazy. She allows group sessions to get out of hand. She relishes bizarre behavior, always keeping it at a safe distance. She maintains order with bone-chilling zeal and establishes an uncomfortable stereotype of nurse as powerful control-freak. She causes the death of one patient and fries the brains of others with electroshock treatment to maintain control. She defeats McMurphy by convincing the medical board that he needs a lobotomy. This restores control within her ward, solidifying her position of power. Nurse Ratched thrives on perfection, order, and obedience. She emasculates male patients while maintaining a sexless facade. Robot-like, she defines the sterile nurse, devoid of human emotion or kindness to the extreme.

Misery (1990), based on Stephen King's book, features another Oscar-winning performance, this time by Kathy Bates, as overweight psychopathic nurse, Annie Wilkes. She is a twisted fan of novelist, Paul Sheldon, played by James Caan. The title is a double entendre as Sheldon's successful series of novels portrays the character Misery Chastain, with whom Wilkes is obsessed and whom Sheldon "kills off" in a later novel. Wilkes finds the writer after a car accident in a snowstorm and takes him home to secretly care for him. She drugs, tortures, and controls him which, in her mind, are noble acts. She is obsessively neat and does not swear. She stockpiles medications, invents orthopedic tools, has romantic fantasies, gets depressed with the rain, and has multiple personalities, one of which is a raging killer. She obsessively ridicules and shames him. This film shows how much power a nurse actually has over her patient. The desire and necessity to trust a nurse can put one's life in peril.

These examples are obviously fictional distortions. But what in these characters rings true? Why can't we forget them? The nurse necessarily must have a bit of aggression and sadism in order to do her job. What about all the needles, poking, prodding, and controlling others' behaviors? Both films leave our jaws agape at the cruelty one human being can inflict on another. The nurse is clearly used as the shadow figure to portray the darker aspects of human nature. It also arouses a sadistic fantasy. Each of these films reverses the pornographer's representation of the female. Rather than begging for domination, this nurse is in control. The reversal of roles shows a woman with power over men.

Sex Object

In the 1970s, a VCR arrived that was affordable and small enough for home use. It spawned a boom in pornography. In pornographic sketches, the nurse is portrayed as naughty, insatiable, and sexually convenient. Why is the nurse the target of pornographic sexual fantasies? Certainly she is not shy about what most people fear—body fluids, sexual organs, and nakedness. Breaking social taboos for the nurse is an everyday occurrence. Pornography is designed for men and 95% of nurses are women, so it is a simple equation. Pornography presents the male fantasy. It shows women submitting to and satisfying men. Pornography has little to do with what brings a woman sexual pleasure. The nurse, guide to the underworld, self-abnegating, and silent, like Hygeia, is titillating prey for the pornographer's lens.

Deep Throat (1972) caught an unsuspecting public by storm and had an impact on every strata of society. Written as a porno comedy with an actual plot, it initially seemed to have a positive impact on expanding sexual curiosities. The story revolves around the film's main character, played by Linda Lovelace, a sexually frustrated woman, who cannot have an orgasm and seeks a physician's help. He discovers her clitoris is in her throat and prescribes stimulating her throat with a penis to achieve orgasm, a quintessential male fantasy. Even better, Lovelace has the prodigious capacity to swallow an entire penis. The humor of *Deep Throat* is built around the general agreement that many women do not relish giving men oral sex, so the idea that this would bring her such pleasure is obviously ironic. The physician's office nurse and casual sex partner is played by Carol Connors and as the film progresses Lovelace also assumes a naughty nurse role.

Deep Throat was a social and commercial phenomena. In a 2005 documentary, *Inside Deep Throat*, Ruth Westheimer, better known as Dr. Ruth, expressed approval that female orgasm was brought up in the film at all, although she reminds us that male fantasy is still the priority of the film. Author Erica Jong commented that, although she was initially enthusiastic about the film, she was quickly disappointed by the later hostile response of the government and the more demeaning porno films modeled on *Deep Throat* that ensued. Jong said that the cynical porn industry took advantage of the first amendment, changing the nature of porn from art to money.

With President Nixon's landslide re-election in 1972, repression and censorship increased. An FBI investigation revealed that half the videos on the market were hard-core pornography and most of the millions of profit from *Deep Throat*, which cost less than $25,000 to make, went to the mob. Pornography became an avenue for voyeurism through home accessibility, and the pornographic nurse fantasy peaked during the "Golden Age of Porn" from the late 1960s through the early 1980s. Rather than promoting knowledge about the body, eros, and sexual liberation, pornography thrived on shame and humiliation. The pornographer reduced woman to pleasure object without need for pleasure herself. I have not met a woman yet who puts anal intercourse or having semen squirted into her eyes at the top of her list for sexual pleasure. These are a male fantasy, plain and simple.

Now, to art. Richard Prince created 42 "Nurse Paintings" in 2003, inspired by covers of cheap pulp fiction novels from the 1950s and 1960s. He focused on consumer culture, simultaneously capturing the erotic and the menacing nurse. These images raise ambivalent feelings about sex, purity, and vulnerability. So irresistible, the paintings sold for a minimum of $5,000,000 each. In these paintings, the nurse wears uniform and cap, is masked, appears bashful, and is slender, with a 1950s hairstyle, thick eye makeup, and grace in the motions of her hand. She plays the part of object of possibility, suggesting danger. The mask covering her mouth often has blood-colored lipstick seeping through—red, the color of life. It sometimes drips down her arms and on her uniform. Since her mouth is covered, she remains anonymous. The nurse's eyes and body say come-hither as well as emit caution. Accessible yet forbidden, available yet out of reach, the nurse is wholesome yet on intimate terms with strangers' bodies. She is alluring, dangerous, and kinky. Each "Nurse Painting" holds the promise of virgin and whore. The nurse's hands clean a man's body, reminding him of his primal animal nature as well as his vulnerability. The nurse as sex object is a deep-seated stereotype.

Major Margaret Houlihan, a highly competent nurse, is tagged with this stereotype in the film, $M*A*S*H$ (1970), based on the novel written by Richard Hooker, pseudonym for surgeon H. Richard Hornberger, and adapted to screen by the author and Ring Lardner, Jr. Under the direction of Robert Altman, we are introduced to the incomparable, "Hot Lips" Houlihan. She was played by Sally Kellerman in the film, and later by Loretta Swit in the wildly popular and enduring television series. Houlihan, described as "fortyish" in the novel, is intelligent and strong with high ethical standards. She has an insatiable libido and personifies one of the favorite nurse images in contemporary culture. Houlihan's clinical competence is indisputable. Hawkeye, surgeon and primary protagonist, describes her as "a pain in the ass but a damn good nurse."

Set in a mobile army surgical hospital, *M*A*S*H* exposes the dark comedic side of war and the gallows humor necessary for survival. Houlihan, a buxom blonde in charge of the army nurses, becomes intimate with a righteous surgeon, Frank Burns. They share sexual rendezvous and berate the other surgeons for their unmilitary-like behavior. A secret microphone in Burns's tent during raucous lovemaking allows the entire camp to hear her say, "Kiss my hot lips," coining her nickname forever. The fact that she is a sexual woman and shows her vulnerability takes precedence over everything else. She never lives it down and remains the butt of the surgeons' irreverent jokes forever.

Often films characterize the sexual fantasy nurse, never showing her on duty. *South Pacific*

(1958), an adaptation of the Rogers and Hammerstein musical, based on James Michener's 1947 book of short stories, *Tales of the South Pacific*, imparts the story of a perky and naïve Ensign Nellie Forbush, played by Mitzi Gaynor, who is romantically involved with a French island plantation owner. The other nurses in *South Pacific* fuel the sexual fantasies of sailors and never show any nursing knowledge or expertise. In *Catch-22* (1970), adapted from Joseph Heller's 1961 novel, wartime nurses with cleavage are shown gossiping, heartless and unmoved, while ignoring patients. One nurse teases her hair while talking to a patient. There's also a fantasy scene with a nurse naked on a water barge. Both films illustrate a very common nurse stereotype—the nurse as shallow eye candy.

Why do nurses play into this stereotype and dress up in sexy costumes for parties? I've done it myself—bunny ears, tail, and all. This is necessary to counter the regulated modesty required by our professional role. In addition we identify with this stereotype so ingrained in popular culture. Dressing up as a sexy nurse for a work party disarms the dominant hierarchy. As Jungian analyst, Marion Woodman, says, "There is nothing stronger than whore energy to depotentiate the patriarchal collective that has kept the virgin silent."

THE NURSE IN POPULAR CULTURE

Angel of Mercy

At the other extreme is the image of the nurse as angel of mercy. In this personification, the nurse is compliant, pure, and dedicated, often with a religious vocation linked to the piety of the Victorian Age. Henry Wadsworth Longfellow's 1857 poem, "Santa Filomena," depicts Florence Nightingale as its exemplar, "A lady with a lamp. . ." In this poem, it is the nurse's shadow darkening walls that the patient wants to kiss, not the noble, all-good, heroic woman. This is interesting because the psychological term "shadow" was not yet commonly used in Longfellow's day to reflect the complexity of unwanted and concealed contents in the unconscious. He makes the nurse one-dimensional and portrays her as a fantasy figure. The angel of mercy remains a devoted servant without needs of her own. It is the saintly and out-of-reach aspects that appeal to Longfellow. In Pisa, Italy, there is a chapel dedicated to Santa Filomena with a picture of her as nymph with angels above the sick and maimed. This mural displays the paradox of the nurse who is both accessible and out of reach.

The first film biography of Florence Nightingale, *The White Angel* (1936), reflects only her virtuous and high-minded side and leaves out the shadow and complexity, not only of Nightingale, but of the nursing profession itself. A film made for television, *Florence Nightingale* (1985), emphasizes that the nurse should be patient and silent, tending to everyone except herself, another common trait that continues today. Today's nurse continues to be self-sacrificing.

Angel of Death

The nurse as psychopomp mediates between life and death and is often personified as the angel of death. In the film, *The English Patient* (1996), based on the novel by Michael Ondaatje, Juliette Binoche, who received an Academy Award for her performance, portrays a battle-worn WWII nurse, Hana, who bonds with a severely burned patient, Count Almasy, played by Ralph Fiennes. They are stationed alone in a dilapidated Italian villa. As he suffers and discloses the intimate details of his life, their relationship intensifies. The devotion she offers him is palpable as her own woundedness comes to the surface. Almasy shares memories of a lover that died. Hana remains compassionate and professional, tending him physically and psychologically while she also is tormented by her own demons. She is generous with morphine to keep him from suffering.

Finally, Almasy pushes all the morphine ampules towards Hana saying with his eyes that he wishes to die. In this pivotal and highly emotional scene, she opens all of the ampules and honors the patient's wishes. As she injects the morphine, she reads to him the love letters left by his dead lover. She smiles when he quietly dies. It was his choice and she supports him with no agenda of her own. She never shies away from her part in the intensely difficult decision and accepts the harsh reality. She is the nurse as psychopomp leading her patient through dark veils and shadows toward death.

Handmaiden

The handmaiden, imaged as silent Hygeia, is a capable and efficient helper. She assists the physician often without using her own judgment, intelligence, or autonomy. She exists merely to help the physician. Deeply ingrained in the collective psyche, she is the woman who assists a man in his aspirations. Her vacant hope is that he will rescue her from loneliness, emptiness, and unrealized dreams.

Mythologist Joseph Campbell distinguishes between the revered and the repulsive girl. He explains that it is the revered Grail maiden who obeys her own heart, whereas the loathsome damsel fails to obey her heart and only follows instructions of others. This is a significant mythological statement that applies to a nurse who does not act from her heart, develops no moral code of her own, and becomes a pawn in the hierarchy of healthcare.

The film, *Awakenings* (1990), based on the 1973 Oliver Sacks memoir, is set in a long-term convalescent home for vegetative patients with brain damage. It serves as a microcosm for a society sedating rather than dealing with the messiness of disease and death. There is one seasoned nurse who dives in to help a new physician implement a study that wakes these patients up with synthetic dopamine, music, literature, and human contact, while the other nurses are watching soap operas without much interest in their unconscious patients.

Once patients begin to wake up, they want more freedom. Chaos ensues and the administrators fear losing control. A parallel example is the Intensive Care Unit (ICU) nurse who is notorious for being most content when her patient is intubated and sedated. The film thoughtfully examines the tendency to defend the status quo rather than enter the messiness of conscious awareness.

Miss Evers' Boys (1997) is an important HBO television film based on a true story, adapted from the 1992 stage play by physician, David Feldshuh. As Eunice Evers, Alfre Woodard plays an African-American nurse complicit in the 1932 Tuskegee study. Like most actual nurses of the era, the nurse never challenges the physician. The film amplifies the tragedy of this point of view. Miss Evers feels it is wrong to withhold penicillin from her patients yet defers authority to the physician. On other occasions, though, she shows her clinical acumen. An example is when a physician is raging at a young boy who has injured himself while climbing a tree. She listens to the boy's chest and subtly suggests in a non-threatening way that there is fluid around his heart. The physician takes her suggestion and asks for a long pericardial needle to pull the fluid off. She saves the boy's life. This is a very common scenario in which the nurse tactfully suggests a remedy overlooked by the physician. The capacity of the nurse is enormous but as handmaiden she is silently obedient.

Eunice Evers follows doctors' orders blindly without question. Not only is she complicit but she also lies and keeps secrets from her dying patients. She tells them they are getting treatment when in reality only data is being collected. The spinal taps have their own risks—infection, bleeding, and herniation. She sanctifies the ethics of obedience. The saddest part is that patients keep coming back because of her kindness, yet she is clearly contributing to catastrophic consequences. The nurse as a passive participant in unethical practice is frightening. Patients are in danger when nurses are oppressed.

Sacrificial Servant

Self-sacrifice is the most universal trait found in all nurses. In ancient times, sacrifice as ritual made daily life sacred. It acknowledged the divinities and the debt owed to nature. Artistic images from the Middle Ages and the Renaissance often portrayed nurses delivering or caring for a baby. Later Christian images portrayed nurses not as family members or servants but attending to domestic, spiritual, and physical care. Nuns who functioned as nurses were not subordinate to physicians. Neither saints nor miracle worker, the nurse was firmly rooted in common activities of day to day life.

The Nun's Story (1959), a film based on the 1956 novel by Kathryn Hulme, illustrates how a nurse puts others' health and safety above her own. Audrey Hepburn plays a passionate novitiate, Gabrielle, who becomes Sister Luke. She leaves her biological father to devote her entire life to God the Father. She dreams of serving in the Congo and she fully commits her life to God and the rules of the convent.

Silence is demanded on the exterior as well as the interior with nonessential conversation forbidden. Interior silence is described as a way to strive for perfection. Each initiate's goal is to make herself invisible and always to be aware of others' needs. Examples of this are closing the door quietly, never asking for anything, and walking close to the wall so as not to take up too much space. Another rule is not to walk too slowly or be in a hurry. The initiate must be attentive, alert, and obedient in all things. The goal of these mandates is to purge her of all passions and faults. Each member keeps a journal of implications in which she confesses all her transgressions. It starts with the statement, "I accuse myself of . . ." The journal is read aloud to the community and followed by penance. Such rigid rules are designed to force the initiate to fully embrace humility. Gabrielle's attempt at perfection takes its toll.

After returning from the Congo to occupied Europe during WWII, Gabrielle can no longer blindly obey her vow of obedience. She courageously breaks rules to help the Resistance. Rebellion is a trait more of the nurse than the nun. The nature of rebellion is to face the enemy within. Once the rebel understands herself, she can follow through authentically. Obedience without question has been Gabrielle's struggle all along. She chooses to be a nurse rather than a nun. As the film ends, she triumphantly leaves her post to work as a nurse in the underground Resistance.

THE SOUL OF THE NURSE

Passion Fish (1992), a film written and directed by John Sayles, stars again Alfre Woodard, this time as Chantelle, a nurse who struggles between work and her personal life. She is a drug addict just out of detox. Her daughter was taken from her and she misses her terribly. Chantelle is the first nurse that a newly paraplegic soap opera star, May-Alice, played by Mary McDonnell, can tolerate because she does not fall for May-Alice's "poor me" victim racket. The film displays a comical smorgasbord of nurse stereotypes—wearing a starched uniform, pushing tranquilizers, being rough with the patient, washing walls obsessively, talking incessantly, crying constantly, star-struck, riding a motorcycle, smoking, and loving bad boys—before these "types" are fired. In the end, Chantelle helps May-Alice stop numbing herself with alcohol and May-Alice supports Chantelle in solidifying her break from addiction and moving toward a reconnection with her daughter. The relationship proves to be transformative for both patient and nurse. Chantelle initially takes the job as penance for her addiction and, through self-sacrifice, helps herself.

Heroine

The heroine displays self-sacrifice but to a greatly magnified degree. She separates herself from her community and goes on a journey with a mission to seek justice. The heroine gives up everything, even her life, on behalf of an ideal. The image of the heroine is likely projected onto the nurse by patients because, when people are ill, they are vulnerable and scared. Rather than fear that the nurse is incompetent or even demonic, they project upon her a role of superiority as Longfellow did with Florence Nightingale.

The ultimate nurse heroine is seen in the film, *So Proudly We Hail* (1943). Shot during World War II and based on actual United States Army Nursing Corps records, eight Red Cross nurses face unpredictability, danger, and death. Joan O'Doul, played by Paulette Goddard, wears a black lace nightie as a dress, attempting to maintain her femininity. Janet "Davy" Davidson, played by Claudette Colbert, falls in love with a soldier and spends her wedding night in a fox hole. Olivia D'Arcy, played by Veronica Lake, is disillusioned and bitter because her lover was killed by the enemy. She wants revenge and fantasizes about becoming a cold-blooded killer, asking to work in the enemy ward. The matronly nurse supervisor is wise to this and transfers her before she can harm any patients. When the nurses are trapped, about to be raped and killed, Olivia puts a live grenade in her bra, lets down her long blonde hair, and seductively walks toward the enemy. The grenade explodes and provides escape for her nurse colleagues. She makes the ultimate sacrifice.

The 2004 remake of the 1978 zombie classic, *Dawn of the Dead*, features heroine Ana Clark, played by Sarah Polley, as the smart, brave, resourceful nurse helping survivors stay alive and literally stay human. She narrowly escapes multiple attacks from the ever-growing number of flesh-seeking zombies. Ana leads the survivors with composure, compassion, and intelligence. She figures out that a zombie bite dooms a human to death to join the walking dead. She is heroic, the ultimate survivor, outsmarting her enemies, caring for the others, and saving them over and over again. The nurse heroine, as depicted in these films, has tremendous courage, demonstrates immense capabilities in a crisis, and takes daring action in situations which most others would avoid.

Matron-Spinster

The hardened matron from the working class is often a senior nurse who is efficient, battle-ready, and worn. She is styleless, without a partner or home-life, and often is self-important in her authority. A well-known nurse figure, dignified with an established position in the hierarchy, she runs a tight ship and is a strict disciplinarian. She wears a starched white uniform, stockings, and cap. Remember, in prehistoric times, white is associated with death. She is naturally feared by all. Paradoxically, the matron is often a guise covering a wild maenad that resides within.

In Baz Luhrmann's film adaptation of Shakespeare's *Romeo and Juliet* (1996), the nurse looks like a frumpy matron but in truth is colorful and multidimensional and plays a crucial role in the story. There is controversy over even the name of this nurse or if she has a name at all. It is conjectured that her name is Angelica, but her name is obscure and only mentioned once in Shakespeare's play. I like the paradoxical link of her name to the stereotype of "angel." Her initial employment is as wet nurse to Juliet, nanny, and servant to the family. She becomes the confidante and guide for Juliet and Romeo. The nameless nurse, like Baubo, offers comic relief and constantly moves the plot forward. We sense there is a maenad under the surface as she brings us down to earth, provokes laughter, showing common bonds while pointing out hypocrisy, imbalance, and absurdities.

Juliet's nurse displays the only feminine nurturing in the household. She is fat, with an unfashionable hairdo, and she revels in romance and love. She serves as messenger and arranges a time for Juliet to meet Romeo at the church for a secret marriage. She is naïve yet wise, irreverent as well as devout, ultimately a fraud and trustworthy—the ultimate paradox.

In the film *The World According to Garp* (1982), based on John Irving's 1978 novel, Glenn Close plays an unconventional matron-spinster nurse, Jenny. She deliberately impregnates herself with an unconscious soldier's erect phallus before he dies because she wants a child without a husband. Like Isis/Hathor, she re-members and uses courage and trickery to regenerate. Certainly, to say the least, she is pragmatic and raises her son with unconventional honesty. She remains practical in her approach to sexuality and adventure.

Jenny runs an infirmary at a private school for boys where, true to character, she is kind but stern. She tells her son Garp all that matters is the adventures one can have in life. When Garp reaches the age of sexual awareness, she initially gets angry and tries to control him. Then she hires a prostitute to teach him the ways of sex. Jenny publishes a book, *Sexual Suspect*, a heretical manifesto about woman as wife or whore and insists the only thing Garp inherited from her was the ability to piss people off. Jenny is peculiar, with the looks of a dignified strict matron from the working class, even in her uniform, yet underneath, we delight in her irreverence.

Rouser of Revelry

The rouser of revelry shocks us by using frank candor and audacity to get a rise out of others. Goethe's *Faust* characterizes Baubo as riding a pig. This image suggests animal-like obscenity rather than the revered nurse that affirms life. Charles Dickens, in his nineteenth-century satire, *Martin Chuzzlewit*, employs harsh humor to display the amusing drunk nurse Mrs. Sarah Gamp, which was an accurate depiction of those working in the role of nurse prior to the Nightingale era. Gamp, from the ranks of the unsophisticated working class, is straightforward, improper, and clearly a rebel. This has validity in mythology, literature, and historical accountings. Despite Gamp's lack of refinement, like Baubo, she is an important and revered figure, even preferred over a more competent nurse, perhaps because of the primitive authenticity she embodies.

In one scene Gamp takes a pinch of snuff, stands over an ill man with her head tilted, stoops down, and pins his arms against his sides saying, "Ah!, he'd make a lovely corpse." This is an excellent example of the gallows humor nurses employ. Ever resourceful, Gamp keeps potential employees from learning too much about her own deplorable behavior by inventing former employers "for the purpose of attesting to her own goodness of heart and beneficence of conduct" and "brightness of her inner light." As nurse, Gamp approaches adversity as ritual. She is common folk close to the earth and to flesh. Her failings are overshadowed by her perseverance and endurance under miserable circumstances. She guides others through unpredictable hardships. Nothing surprises her because she has witnessed so much human folly and suffering.

My favorite illustration of the rouser of revelry comes from the Showtime series, *Nurse Jackie*. A former nurse colleague, whom Jackie refers to as the "bitch-on-wheels," arrives in the emergency room with advanced cancer. She knows her colleagues are the only ones that will carry out her wishes to die. Knowingly breaking the law, each staff member contributes supplies of morphine until there is enough accumulated to euthanize her. The entire staff gathers around the patient's gurney with champagne as the morphine is pushed into the intravenous line. With typical crusty nurse gallows humor, the "bitch-on-wheels" says, "Fuck you and here's to me," then dies. The irreverent scene is a realistic portrayal of how the majority of nurses feel and what they would do if euthanasia were legal.

Another scene I can't leave out is in the 1981 film, *Whose Life is it Anyway?* Here, paralyzed Ken Harrison, played by Richard Dreyfus, wants to die and the physicians refuse to allow it, saying, "Death is the enemy," and that it is their duty to prolong life. To keep him quiet, they give him unwanted tranquilizers. Ken sues and eventually wins his trial based on habeas corpus and illegal imprisonment and will be allowed to die. An orderly, played by Thomas Carter, tucks him into bed and pulls the sheet over his face as if he were dead. Both shake with uncontrollable laughter. Sometimes laughing at the absurd is the only thing that can make us sane.

Demon-Lover

The nurse often falls for the outcast or rebel due to her non-judgmental attitude and need for excitement. She desires to rescue others and lusts for partners who engage in risk. Nurses helping criminals and falling in love with a bad boy are portrayed in films like *Prison Nurse* and *Night Nurse. Prison Nurse* (1938), set in a state prison that is flooding, opens with no physicians available. Three nurses volunteer and brave the rising waters to make their way into the prison to help. One of the prisoners is a physician but refuses to help until he is compelled to do so after a man is shot. The nurses save the day, and one of them falls in love with the physician-prisoner. The attraction of the demon-lover is his intensity and the thrill of his unpredictable behavior. He has a youthful demeanor, like a teenager, and thus has a vulnerable quality that is irresistible to a nurse. He, too, is familiar with living on the edge, near death. *Night Nurse* has the demon-lover leitmotif as well, and will be discussed next.

Multidimensional Nurse Characters

Before censorship guidelines were enforced in 1934, Pre-Code films often included hints of sex, villainous characters who profited from their exploits, and strong heroic women as main characters. *Night Nurse* (1931) reveals the raw nature of the nursing profession. Barbara Stanwyck plays Lora Hart, a woman with street-smarts. After being told by the unfriendly nursing supervisor that she does not quality for the hospital nurse training program, she bumps into the top medical officer who takes a liking to her immediately. He takes her to the strict matron who didn't realize Lora "knew" this important figure and she is immediately enrolled. Lora's savvy charm gets her in the door, and she is unaffected by the nursing supervisor's attempt at intimidation.

A sisterhood develops between Lora and another trainee, B. Maloney, played by Joan

Blondell, as they recognize one another from their origins of poverty. With similar values and ideals, they are tough and can handle getting pushed around by thugs, behavior displayed as normal for nurses in this film. The two display opposites in sincerity and sarcasm while reciting the Nightingale pledge. Lora is moved while B. is bored and chewing gum. The scenes of the nurses undressing may symbolize the naked truth as illusions of an altruistic profession are stripped away. B. works days, and Lora nights, holding opposite ends of the archetype. Lora exposes two men trying to murder her patients and steal their inheritance. Both nurses abandon the nursing pledge of confidentiality in order to speak out and seek justice.

Night Nurse portrays the personal, educational, and bureaucratic challenges nurses face. It displays that telling the truth and seeking justice is no easy task. The nurse is truly a moral leader. Lora protects the innocent and breaks the rules in order to protect her patients. She accepts the dark side of human beings and has a weakness for the demon-lover. Lora is less educated than the physicians yet she is wiser, more clever, and has a more humane value system. She has a nose for hypocrisy, fights tenaciously against red tape, and demonstrates what an idealistic new nurse is capable of accomplishing.

THE SOUL OF THE NURSE

The sisterhood of nursing is beautifully portrayed in *Night Nurse* because it shows mutual support of values, and nurses covering for one another and living together. The film illustrates the fundamental virtues of teamwork and relationship. The film sadly shows the degree to which nurses are beaten down by bureaucracy and how they are oppressed by the hierarchy within nursing as well as by physicians and administrators. Ethics during this era was understood within the profession as obedience to authority. When Lora breaks her silence about a rape she witnessed, she is fired. Even the best, seemingly most moral physician tries to convince her not to testify, arguing that it would give her the reputation as a meddler. She is banned from nursing for speaking out and accepts a marriage proposal from a bootlegger who is a former patient she treated for a gun shot wound. The film ends as she leaves her career behind to marry the bad boy.

Another excellent illustration of a multidimensional nurse figure occurs in the film, *Wit* (2001), adapted from a one-act play by Margaret Edson, which takes place in a university hospital and explores a patient's experience of illness while exposing the lack of humanity in medical research. Vivian Bearing, played by Emma Thompson, is intelligent yet helpless and unskilled as a patient. She is single with no friend or advocate. She has done little contemplation about her own death. An English scholar and literature professor, she recites fervently John Donne's Holy Sonnet X, "Death, be not proud," throughout her diagnosis and treatment for Stage IV ovarian cancer.

A detached research physician, played by Christopher Lloyd, convinces Vivian to undergo an aggressive chemotherapy research protocol that offers slim chance of survival. She is swayed to participate due to their shared pride in academic research. She unwittingly participates in the brutal experiment. As her condition deteriorates and her fears increase, nurse Susie Monahan, played by Audra McDonald, gives Vivian honest, professional nursing care with integrity and depth. Susie clashes with the physicians and opposes the chemotherapy protocol. The cruel indifference toward Vivian shown by physicians is countered by Susie's kindness. Susie is steady and conveys straight forward honesty. Vivian comes to trust Susie, which has a significant impact on Vivian's emotional, spiritual, and physical health. At the end of the film, despite Vivian's wishes to allow natural death, when she codes, the medical team pounces on her with cardiopulmonary resuscitation. Susie prevents the medical team from carrying it out by putting her own body between the team and the patient and prevents more torture and indignity.

Angels in America (2003), a six part HBO television series, gives us one of the most authentic nurses in film, Belize, played by Emmy- and Golden Globe-winner Jeffrey Wright. Belize is an African-American gay nurse who cares for Roy Cohn, played by Al Pacino. Cohn is a powerful lawyer in denial of his homosexuality, AIDS diagnosis, and mortality. He is loathed by the gay community for his hypocrisy. Despite Cohn's reputation, Belize treats him with candor and dignity. When Belize is told that the new patient is a "very important man," he responds sarcastically about being sure he won't mess up his medications.

By far, Belize is the most compassionate and decent person in the film, albeit embittered by the lack of universal access to treatment for AIDS. Cohn asks Belize if he is here to escort him to the underworld and indeed Belize is present when he dies. Displaying expertise in post-mortem care, Belize calls on his Jewish friend to recite the Kaddish after Cohn's death, showing how nurses honor the varied cultural and religious beliefs of patients. Belize then absconds with Cohn's stockpile of AZT for distribution to his afflicted friends who don't have access to the medication. This again is the nurse circumventing an unjust system, doing what it takes to help others in need.

Nurse Jackie (2009 - 2012) is a television first—a show with a realistic, multi-layered nurse as the main character. The protagonist, Jackie Peyton, played by Edie Falco, is dealing with personal issues of pain, denial, addiction, and ultimately her underlying existential alienation. Her very human character shows that genuine nursing care is not given by angelic handmaidens or sex objects. Most hospital nurses enjoy the rush of adrenaline as well as the constant opportunity to help and rescue others. The series exaggerates and brings to the surface repressed and denied parts of Jackie in the safe container of fiction.

The trailer introduces Jackie lying on the floor in a white starched uniform and cap, in a dream state, reciting T. S. Eliot's "The Love Song of J. Alfred Prufrock"—"Let us go then, you and I/When the evening is spread out against the sky/Like a patient etherized upon a table." Jackie is scheming, proficient, and smart. Her hard exterior is countered by her soft heart. She displays the nurse's ability to work the system. She even convinces insurance companies to cover procedures normally denied. In a departure from the expected heroine nurse figure, she is an addict and her addiction dominates everything, putting her at a distance from everyone in her life and shows how demoralized many nurses are today. She has no friends outside of work. She is neither gloomy nor cheery and looks for escape through substances. To make the series more seductive, she has sex with a pharmacist while on the job in return for drugs. Yet she remains a consummate professional in her work as well as a struggling wife and mother.

As nurse, central to patient care, Jackie is the one who knows what is happening in the hospital. She shares a quote she heard from a nun in nursing school. "The people with the greatest capacity for good are the ones with the greatest capacity for evil." She retorts, "Smart fucking nun." This is similar to the C. S. Lewis concept that the devil is at work wherever we are doing good. She has back pain, a common work injury symptom of the nurse. She snarls, "What do you call a nurse with a bad back? Answer: Unemployed."

Jackie attacks the new physician, Coop, played by Peter Fucinelli, when he dismisses her suggestion that a brain scan should be done and the patient dies because he fails to order it. In response, Coop grabs Jackie's breast, claiming to have a Tourettes-type reaction to anxiety, displaying, in Hollywood fashion, the sexual harassment that occurs in the work place. Jackie doesn't make much of it, accepting it as part of a day's work.

In another scene, Jackie tells the peppy, talkative student nurse, Zoey Barkow, played by Merritt Wever, who wears childish scrubs with matching earrings, that she likes her protégées to be quiet and mean. Jackie's elegant female physician friend, Eleanor O'Hara, played by Eve Best, tells Jackie she is the only sane one and explains that physicians are into cutting up animals in science class while nurses are into healing, helping, and fixing.

Interestingly, some nursing organizations wanted a disclaimer suggesting *Nurse Jackie* does not portray a real nurse. In my estimation, Falco's virtuoso portrayal of a nurse is the best since Barbara Stanwick's Lora Hart or Jeffrey Wright's Belize. We can only hope to find nurses with Jackie's empathy, skill, and consistency in standing up for patients. She has softness and compassion under the hard shell often developed in the profession. Her manipulation and calculating approach is a sign that something is terribly amiss in healthcare. She is imperfect, human, and the kind of nurse I want when I am sick.

Being invisible is both a desire and a curse. A deeper look at Jackie's sex and drug habit begs the question, what is the allure of drugs and sex for nurses? Is there some truth to the nurse needing to find spirit in a spiritually bleak environment? Is this an attempt at re-connection with the body? What is behind the underlying sadness, distance, and lack of intimacy? Although Jackie shows just how unfailingly she deceives everyone, she really is alienated and in trouble because of her life-long self-deception. Tension builds as we wonder how this excellent nurse will ever find self-fulfillment while continuing to give so much to her patients.

Jackie takes care of the vulnerable, usually without getting confused by her own agenda, until her addiction gets in the way. She begins to be confronted. She is absent from her children. She is jealous of her husband's peace of mind because he can sleep at night. She shows pain, loneliness, and fear of losing the man that loves her. Her friend O'Hara jokingly tells Jackie, "You're awful." And in comic fashion she responds, "That's what I'm trying to tell you." She is desperate as she grasps at quick fixes that take her further and further away from experiencing true self-love and groundedness.

Jackie has the ability to influence the collective image of nursing. *Nurse Jackie* also makes every nurse look more deeply at herself and her behavior while highlighting pertinent issues in nursing and healthcare such as end of life care, dangerous breakdowns in communication between medicine and nursing, and the importance of giving the nurse a voice. *Nurse Jackie* entertains, refutes stereotypes, and keeps it real. Perhaps *Nurse Jackie* is showing just how broken-hearted the nurse is today, unable to provide safe, effective, dignified care to each patient due to a healthcare system that needs re-imagining.

Popular culture teaches us that the nurse is relentless. She gets the job done. She is a rebel seeking justice and equality for her patients; she breaks rules if she feels it will benefit her patient. She attempts to remain invisible while manipulating the system. She revels in love and sex and is a compulsive perfectionist and control freak. She is lonely, seeking embodied spirit, countering with humility, courage, and compassion. She denies herself work breaks and time off. She is practical and down to earth and not a miracle worker. She understands and accepts the cycle of life and attempts the best she can to alleviate suffering.

Medicine today is practiced at a distance, as if looking at a battle like a general from afar. Nurses are engaged on the front line, directly in contact with the ill. They are vulnerable, as are their patients. The work is close and involved. Rather than a contract ensuring patient compliance, perhaps a more secure covenant is needed between patient and nurse, an agreement linking the nurse-patient in a bond, each understanding who the other really is.

CHAPTER 5
Finding the Soul of the Nurse

Imagination, inner work, sensations of the body, and dreams awaken the soul. The common legacy shared by all nurses provides a collective bond. For the nurse, real soul work is about exploring her own adversity, not avoiding melancholy but entering her depths in order to meet what her soul craves. Symbols and metaphors provide helpful tools for excavating what is below the surface. The nurse, by re-membering her personal and collective stories, can transform her life. The mythological approach shifts from linear and limited thinking to ambiguous and complex awareness.

To make whole does not mean to make perfect or normal. Rather it opens the nurse's personal capacity so she has more access to her entire being. Scary and strange dreams give clues to what the soul craves. Soul is activated by images that are disfigured, bizarre, and obscene. The courage to face what is peculiar and flawed defines the nurse's character.

Self-Discovery

Impulses, feelings, and beliefs deemed unacceptable are not permitted into conscious awareness. To look at the shadow is to intentionally address what is hidden. The shadow refers to anything good or bad, repressed or denied. The shadow most often implies the parts of the psyche that are most despised, feared, and rejected. The soul is drawn to these dark and untidy places. Paradoxically, repressing one's talents is as damaging as suppressing the unappealing aspects of personality. When I started working on this book, initially I was drawn to dark and peculiar aspects of the nurse. For me, dark shadow areas were more accessible and easier to acknowledge. In time it registered that the positive is more difficult to fully accept.

Becoming conscious of repressed characteristics is the only way the nurse can avoid repeating old patterns and behaviors. Sharing these split-off pieces with others can bring delight, acceptance, and camaraderie. Sharing, at the very least, adds another perspective. Entering into what feels like dangerous territory, inviting and provoking uncomfortable emotions, breaks down boundaries and limitations.

As for the maenad, unbridled expression of body sensations linked to personal suffering and ecstasy are necessary for the re-imagination of the soul of the nurse. While it is necessary to explore the sustaining images of the nurse, the essence of soul work is to uncover what is individually highly sensitive and personal. It is the particulars that reveal the universal. Morality is not the concern in the process and that is why mythology is so helpful in unraveling unconscious beliefs that may lead to self-defeating behaviors.

What is hidden in the unconscious keeps the nurse from accounting for behavior like aggression and compulsivity which show up as sabotage, manipulation, and workaholism. Desires and neediness are difficult to admit and often met with guilt and shame. In addition, a nurse who is reluctant to acknowledge her strengths does a disservice as nobody benefits when the talents of a nurse are denied. Anything of substance casts a shadow. The larger something is, the longer is its shadow. Shadow work is essential for self-discovery.

Projections

It is easier to project denied aspects onto others than to admit our own. An example of this is when we insist that someone is either friendly or malicious but cannot be both. We often project our most hated parts onto our so-called enemies when really it is ourselves we need to face. The nurse can also be the scapegoat for anger and other shadow projections from physicians, colleagues, and patients, all of which may adversely affect her.

Suppressed and rejected aspects reside in the unconscious and leak out in impulsive behaviors. This is often seen with preachers and politicians, who clearly don't connect on a meaningful level with their authentic motives, preferences, and beliefs. They claim "family values" only to be caught in a predictable aberrant act and their covert life surfaces in the media.

Anxiety and Complexes

When life seems unmanageable, people attempt to create a world that is orderly without surprises. Since anxiety seems to decrease boredom and increase sharpness, the nurse often feeds anxiety with caffeine and sugar. Jackie illustrates this as she adds uppers and downers in her attempt to cope. Worry and conflict come from the inability to creatively apply stored energy and adapt to new conditions. Rationalization or will power can suppress anxiety and provide short-term relief, but anxiety, with the right trigger, always comes back in its original strength and makes one feel as if someone or something else is to blame. Children lose control and flail their hands and feet in frustration. This is called a tantrum. In adults it is called a complex—an expression of the unconscious part of the psyche. This kind of "acting out" is frequently encountered by the nurse. Strongly emotional, mostly unconscious, a complex has its own autonomy, intention, and value, and pulls its victim into compulsive thinking and actions. C.G. Jung said that we think we have complexes but in truth they have us. The only way to work out a complex is to acknowledge it.

The Wounded Healer

The wounded healer is not simply someone who has a medical history. She is someone on the inside who speaks both the nurse and patient languages fluently because she shares the common experience of illness. As Susan Sontag wrote, "Everyone who is born holds dual citizenship in the kingdom of the well and in the kingdom of the sick." The wounded healer fully embraces disfigurement and suffering because she has lived it. Hecate and nurses in *The English Patient*, *Passion Fish*, and *So Proudly We Hail* are all good examples of wounded healers, who can be present and tolerate intensity with others due to their personal history.

The wounded-healer nurse does not split the patient-nurse archetype. She is constantly learning from her patients. It is a matter of give and take. The patient's struggles mirror her own. She works knowing she is both patient and nurse—both wounded and healer. "Healers," who deny they are wounded, foster a one-sided hierarchy of dominance and control, as seen in the extremes like Nurse Ratched and Annie Wilkes. It places the burden of illness on the patient and the liability of making them well on the nurse, which is counter-productive because healing comes from within. The wounded healer does not make whole, integrate, or put the wounded person back together again. She holds conscious space and acknowledges and meets dismemberment on an intimate and genuine level. Under the best conditions, it is a shared experience.

Detachment and Dissociation

Some connect nursing to mothering, and it is important to make a distinction. The women who raised Dionysus were not mothers but nurses. The mother's duty is to her child while the nurse is committed to her patient. The mother is connected by personal history. She is concerned with the destiny of the child. The nurse, by the nature of the relationship, remains detached. The nurse witnesses the patient's suffering but does not personalize it. She maintains a broader perspective.

In nursing a certain kind of detachment is necessary. When nurses are traumatized over and over, naturally they move toward self-preservation. Detachment allows the nurse to protect herself against over-involvement and repeated trauma. Dissociation shows up as a disconnect between feelings, sensation, cognition, and imagination. Outward signs may be seen as inappropriate jocularity, flip statements of false reassurance, obsession with tasks, and displaced anger. Dissociation quickly leads to burn-out, guilt, and ultimately dissatisfied nurses and patients. There is a fine line between detachment and dissociation of which each nurse must be keenly aware. Otherwise she will alienate herself from her body, pleasure, and loving relationships in her personal life.

Extremes of Passion

Apollo has been quite successful in oppressing the power of the female. Unlucky with women, he clearly hates them, going so far as to claim a woman is unnecessary for childbirth. The Apollonian assault on the nurse has distorted her altruistic calling. She is diminished when labeled timid angel or stoic matron because she is really quite passionate and has needs of her own. If she expresses aggression or libidinal desire, like Hot Lips Houlihan, she is trivialized or ridiculed. Compounding the problem, the nurse's predecessors were not initiated into their full feminine power either.

THE SOUL OF THE NURSE

Rage is an emotion that comes out of loss, betrayal, and injustice. Rage can be a useful tool and needs direction. Calming and appeasing snuff out the passion. Somatic symptoms like headaches, backaches, stomach and intestine problems are treated with medications. Martyrdom, asceticism, and over-identification with duty merely mask indwelling anger. Compulsive shopping and spending consumes energy and time. Some nurses, like Ratched, provoke rage in order to watch others act out what is really going on inside of them. None of these approaches address the underlying problem.

The Dionysian maenad nurse is liberated into her instinctual realm where she can access her life force and take action in the world. This is the call to action Nightingale was talking about to break the chains of inertia and idleness in Victorian women. There is a wanting and waning hope in the maenad's heart. We feel the necessity of her overwhelming turmoil and confusion. Her enthusiasm awakens her passion. Her destructiveness is necessary for innovation and change. Rage is the force that leads to change. As we learn from mythic figures such as Hecate, the Erinyes, the furies, and the maenads, rage is an energy that shakes things up and demands justice.

FINDING THE SOUL OF THE NURSE

The term hysteria, a diagnosis in Nightingale's era, is no longer used as a clinical diagnosis. We've gotten rid of the patriarchal label and, along with it, the call for justice and equality. Women have not assimilated the fury and therefore it comes out in other ways. Women are told repeatedly not to be over-emotional, frantic, or out-of-control. It is unacceptable. Strong feelings, commitment, and fervor are labeled obsessive. Every woman has learned that it is not safe to appear too big or to show passionate feelings. The result is that women lose connection to their natural highs and lows. Many women are deprived of the ability to feel anything at all. Suppression of emotion silences women and binds them to the past.

The early study of the unconscious began with the treatment of Victorian women with hysteria. Rather than approaching hysteria through Dionysian consciousness, early treatments looked to Apollo for cures. Hysteria was linked to sexual deprivation in passionate women, so the treatment was to stimulate genitalia for orgasm by intercourse for married women and massage of the vulva by the midwife or physician for the unwed. Other treatments were bed rest, bland food, seclusion, and sensory deprivation. The soul wants intensity, not relaxation, and these Apollonian reductive treatments suppress rather than release.

When I was growing up, my mother made it clear that sad and angry feelings were not okay. She used to repeat the motto of her alma mater, an all-women's college, "Remember who you are and what you represent," which to me meant be a good girl, don't have any needs, and certainly don't embarrass her. So for me, as for many girls, I could either obey and identify with my mother, or disobey and do anything to avoid being like her. The problem with either is that I couldn't develop my own value system. Living by principles such as "Remember who you are and what you represent" is not living your own life. Of course, many of us choose to follow others' precepts rather than figuring out who we really are. However, living by others' standards always feels unsatisfactory and fake. Developing one's own value system requires trying on different personas, an awkward pursuit that draws push-back before one is sure of any genuine stance.

I often wonder, since so many nurses are diagnosed with depression, if they are outraged against real injustice. And since so many nurses are treated—or placated—with medication, I question what happens to that healthy and helpful melancholy that is actually speaking to legitimate fears, displacement, and loss.

Melancholy used to be known as a necessary creative state. Now, the heavy-hearted mood shows up as irritation and annoyance. We miss the clue that there is legitimate cause. Without entering the emotion, there is only agitation and disconnection from feelings. Expressive women are disparaged. Melancholy demands attention and rage needs outward expression.

Tears are necessary to release pent-up emotional steam. Nurses don't, and often can't, cry. The nun remains a big part of the nurse archetype and nurses maintain some of her tendencies. I had a nun as an instructor for one of my clinical rotations. When I began to tear up, moved by a patient's horrific situation, she pulled me into an alcove. She scolded and scared me and told me I could never be seen crying on the nursing unit because people would lose confidence in me. She was the only person who ever verbalized this unwritten rule, which has certainly been confirmed in more subtle ways throughout the years. In fairy tales like *Rapunzel* and the *Handless Maiden*, and in the myth of *Psyche and Eros*, tears are deemed to be healing.

Choosing to be a maenad is less destructive than resisting. The maenad feeds the spirit. Dionysus evokes the potential desire in the nurse to fuse with the wilds. Perhaps the nurse's tendency toward compulsions is her attempt to resist Dionysus. Today there is a warped illusion of balance and moderation, suggesting that anything that is not balanced is unhealthy or weak. The melancholic maenad nurse has a natural temperament of extremes. Her pensiveness is countered by excess fervor. Balance suggests that perfection is attainable and that there is such a thing as normal. Neither can be found in human reality. Still, therapists and self-help experts try to restore us to balance through moderation. How boring! The nurse holds the ambiguity of extremes.

Naughty and Audacious

The generous female body with pendulous breasts, fleshy buttocks, and rotund belly is well-represented in Neolithic artifacts. Baubo, too displays this powerful vitality. In a word, Baubo is Rabelaisian, a term that refers to the French humorist and satirist of the 16th century who used gross humor to the extreme. She is bawdy, naughty, and capricious. She rejects rationality and intellect. She turns a deaf ear to power and authority. She is blunt. You know what she likes and dislikes. She is neither intimidated nor intimidating. Baubo-like nurses have incredible intuition and don't mind being seen as fools. Baubo is in service of Aphrodite. She displays how much there is to re-member about sexual attitudes as they relate to the nurse.

Baubo's skirt-raising, vulva-exposing gesture symbolizes the awe of sexual pleasure and procreative powers that prevail over death.

As the only girl on horseback working on a cattle ranch, I learned early that swearing and cursing as loud and as often as necessary was perfectly all right. My father explained that it was ranch talk and it was never repeated outside of that setting. All of us cursed frequently while working on the ranch. It was an acceptable way to express frustration and humor and seemed to work magic at moving cattle. Nurses use profanity and humor amongst themselves in a similar way. I have been known to be blunt and swear during times of tension on the nursing unit or to break the tension in a high-level administrative meeting.

Rouser of Revelry

Nurses are experts at using gallows humor to rip away illusion. Contemporary nurse characters like Belize and Jackie come from the same working class background. They have no tolerance for carelessness. They counter their own need for perfection with vigilance and wit. They work hard and play hard, fully engaged in naughty and willful behavior. There is humility and a natural self-effacement because they know there is a potential crisis lurking around every corner.

Looking at what the nurse finds funny says a lot about her. Baubo, Gamp, Belize, and Jackie constantly display gallows humor, which often exposes repressed sadism. The nurse's quick wit, often unrefined, demonstrates that the nurse is in touch with the shadow. Inappropriate laughter at truly horrendous situations releases fear and anxiety. Laughter diminishes self-consciousness, lowers inhibitions, and frees trapped energy.

Virgin Daughter

The original meaning of the word virgin is a woman who belongs to herself without influence or dependency. She has no need to please or be liked. She remains uncontaminated. This is rare in a nurse today because daughters have not been encouraged to be independent, direct, and rebellious. Instead they learn indirect techniques to get what they want while giving the impression they are dependent and helpless. In the film *Miss Evers' Boys*, we see how nurses adapt to men by being charming. They have no identity and become a mirror to a man's reaction. Some nurses are programmed to rely on men to determine their own personality and they work in a setting that requires constant approval from a male hierarchy. The nurse is permeable and thus contaminated by others. Yet it is the nurse's virginal altruism that drives her practice and makes her willing to attend to the woundedness of strangers. She cares for people who are emotionally stripped, irrational, and fighting for survival. She is linked to sexuality, yet she is not a playgirl or Barbie doll. She develops inner masculine traits to support her feminine experience in caring for the ill.

Dreams

The soul longs for intensity and we see this in our bizarre and sometimes nightmarish dreams. As we know, the nurse is willing to go to extremes. She does not remain in the middle. This intense dedication often feels like madness. The conscious mind holds very little. Dream images are expansive and can bring rich messages from the soul. While researching this chapter I had the following dream:

I'm working in a big urban medical center. There is a man who is having his leg amputated and he needs a prosthetic leg before the operation is done. I need to go in a helicopter across the street to pick up his prosthetic leg and bring it back for him. My beeper goes off when I arrive at the other hospital and it is the lab saying the patient's cardiac enzymes are elevated which means he is having a heart attack. So, instead of getting his prosthesis, I go to the pharmacy to get TNK (tenecteplase), a clot buster, fly back to the other hospital, and take it to his nurses to administer.

Then I realize I do not have his prosthetic leg, so I go back to the helicopter pilots and say, "I need to get back over there." I don't understand why I can't just drive over and get it, but I guess it is really busy, so I have to take the helicopter again. The male pilots are in a travel agency and I can tell they don't remember me, even though they just flew me back and forth. They want to sell me something. They work on the computer and tell me it will cost me $4000.00. A nurse manager helps explain my situation and they say, "Fine, it will be $417.00." I'm not sure the money will be approved by the hospital, so I'm in a bind because I was sent to get his leg but came back with a medication to save his life. I made the right decision because I saved his life, but how am I going to get the prosthetic leg that he needs and not have to pay for it out of my own pocket?

My dream revealed to me that the nurse knows the patient needs the medication for his heart. A new leg will do him no good if he dies. The nurse isn't grounded and is flying around up above everything else tending to many tasks. It is difficult to do the right thing without authorization from the powerful bureaucracy.

This makes the nurse feel insecure and doubt herself.

A disabled man in a woman's dream could be interpreted to mean that her masculine aspect is crippled. The nurse is trying to help a man who doesn't have a leg to stand on—he can't hold himself up. The pattern is, the nurse saves his life and helps him get a leg up. The nurse has to fly in a helicopter, which represents spirit—out of body, away from the earth. The work of the feminine is of the earth. She is flying, getting up high where she thinks about how she is going to fix things, much as Apollo views things from afar.

In the process, the feminine is neglected and not even recognized by the helicopter pilots. Like Iphigenia and Cassandra, she is brushed aside. While she is making sure a man can stand on his own two feet and his heart is taken care of, she is disregarded. She saved his life yet she is anxious that the hospital is angry with her. He was having a heart attack and, because she has a good relationship with the lab personnel, they knew to page her with the abnormal lab value. Even though she did the right thing, she might not be reimbursed and might have to pay for his limb. This is a no-win situation. She needs to be recognized for doing good work. The dream tells me that putting the masculine first does not work.

As the the only girl in a large patriarchal family I often felt like an object. I felt disregarded and confused as to why nobody would listen to me at the dinner table. Ironically, my parents publicly preached liberal values. My mother started the local branch of the League of Women Voters, which my father attended, claiming it was the only intelligent meeting in town. I did not realize the impact my male-favored ancestry carried into my contemporary reality. Clearly, I never felt valued as an individual.

The dream posed the question, "How can the nurse be taken seriously so her feminine voice is heard?" First, she cannot hover around above everything. Her script is often, "I'm doing all the right things, why don't I get acknowledgement?" The feminine must be grounded.

The Nurse in Collusion with Patriarchy

A woman who has succeeded in the modern world is often a father's daughter. Even if a nurse does not consider herself a father's daughter, she is a daughter of patriarchy, and thus likely to have similar traits. Also, a nurse raised by a masculine mother, not in touch with her feminine feeling values, will often reject the feminine. This kind of mother uses power rather than love in raising her children. She has co-opted patriarchal ideals and never fully taken up residency in her female body. She sides with power, dominance, and control over relationship, nurturance, and cooperation.

The nurse starts out early in her career, and certainly long before she is a nurse, with distorted thinking due to the pervasive male power principle. I bought into this ethos. I made elaborate family trees and histories of my paternal side but not a word was spent on my maternal ancestry. It was as if the maternal side didn't exist.

A nurse who has accommodated to a masculine-oriented society has rejected her feminine instincts. Successful as she may be, there is a deep sadness and sense of personal failure since she is supporting an external ideal she can never become. Being fully masculine is unattainable for a woman. She becomes "nice" and manipulative, and a workaholic. She has learned which feelings to deny according to authoritative feedback. Full of *shoulds* and *oughts*, she is alienated from her natural center. She is dissociated from dream images and cut off from her body. She rarely experiences rage, lust, or ecstasy.

I heard a rumor from a family friend that my mother suffered a nervous breakdown shortly after giving up her first teaching job. A few days before my mother died, she told me that my father wrote her resignation letter. She simply signed it and put it reluctantly in the mail. She abandoned her first job near the coast and moved to the small agricultural town where his cattle ranch was located. In that era, it was common that a woman's goal was to have a prince sweep her off her feet with a promise of riches and security. My mother ended up with repressed desires and frustrations reflected in her body. She married, had five babies quickly, the first two only 11 months apart. She built a stylish home to her specifications with an architect, became one of the best cooks in town, and was known for her lavish parties. I'm sure this looked enviable from the outside. Yet she was not grounded in the feminine and only after her last child was born did she fully return to her career.

The nurse raised by a mother who is impatient, values efficiency above all, and does not allow for weakness or feelings experiences herself as a thing to be manipulated. I always felt confused, attempting to please my mother, not realizing her perfection standards lacked wisdom. It took a long time to develop an inner perspective of my own.

Because my mother rejected the feminine I did also. I was a tomboy and only showed interest in sports and working on the ranch with my father. Since I was raised without a feminine embodied experience, my genuine inner preferences were distorted. My mother feared and denied her instinctual nature and passed on the same body split to me. Instead of healthy mirroring which would allow me to develop a healthy relationship with myself, I fostered masculine attributes—much like in my dream. I left home early to escape her harmful influence, which saved my life, but injured my heart. The mother-daughter connection represents the ebb and flow of life and, even though splitting off from the mother may be necessary, it creates a wound.

Confronting the mother-daughter relationship takes painful slow work because loyalty is mistaken for love. I was loyal until my mother died, even though this loyalty, which I thought was love, was destroying me. The sad reality was that I had to loathe myself in order to show that I loved and obeyed her. After her death I began to accept and appreciate her, knowing she too carried ancestral wounds. I continue to work on releasing the negative aspects and am learning how to fully inhabit my female body, discovering that my body is not just a source of pain but of pleasure and joy.

Most of the growing up I have done occurred after my mother's death. Dream images of the Black Madonna showed up. Gimbutas links the pre-historic Madonna to the nurse. With dark skin and round generous body, she has obviously been through the fire, holding enormous capacity for love and understanding. With help from women friends, I found that I could evolve and more fully embody the feminine. The mother in my dreams loves me as outcast, as abandoned daughter, and rejoices in my orphan state. She teaches me that my whole life has been a training in the ways of Apollo and orphan mythology. Rather than denigrate and demean, I can reach out to others. The nurse who can come out from under perfection standards will be liberated.

Heroine Without Needs

The nurse must be tough and particularly hardy to endure her difficult work. Jung considered Florence Nightingale a symbol of virtue and feminine heroism. The heroine is certainly part of the nurse archetype, but virtue isn't enough. Heroism easily moves into martyrdom. Chaos is familiar to the nurse. Thus the hospital is a comfortable place to work. She overcommits and habitually says "yes." Her employers are more than happy to take advantage. There is always overtime, work on holidays, weekends, and nights. She also takes over in the family because she feels that no one else is fully competent—too many disasters happen if she is not in charge. She has tried that and always has to clean up the mess. It's easier to do it herself.

The nurse often has a chaotic personal life, taking care of children, parents, in-laws, and many other people. She works long hours, takes no breaks, and in her mind she is indispensable and irreplaceable. It feels as if she will never get caught up, never do enough. She is unfamiliar with down-time, relaxation, and a moment to acknowledge her inner needs. The darker element of the heroine is her delusion of omnipotence. She is intoxicated by her unlimited power and invincibility.

As a matter of course, the nurse at some point in her career becomes overworked. Some lose the meaning of her initial call or over-identify with her nursing role. Over-identifying keeps a nurse from checking in with herself. She is obviously good at working in critical and emergency settings, yet this distracts her from what is going on inside herself. She perseveres but at what cost? She often ignores her health and accrues a number of bodily symptoms. She disguises sadness with anger and loneliness with workaholism. She adds overtime and extra shifts to avoid these feelings. Rarely does she express her own needs and limitations. Valuable aspects of her personality are stifled.

There is nothing wrong with persona. It is part of being a professional. However, when the nurse is not conscious of it, she becomes hollow, overly conscientious, and self-sacrificing to a point of martyrdom. It is appropriate for a nurse not to express her personal feelings. She must put her patient first. Yet, when this spills over into her personal life, it leads to loneliness. Being passionate about work is healthy only when it feeds the soul.

Sacrifice and the Body

Euripides' play, *Iphigenia in Aulis*, dramatizes how patriarchal cultures sacrifice daughters in order to gain political power and glory. In the story, Agamemnon must sacrifice his daughter, Iphigenia, if he wants the winds to take his ships to Troy. Iphigenia refuses to accept that she has been cast off and disregarded by her father. Rather, she blames Helen, the unfaithful wife of Menelaus, for corrupting the social order. In a dramatic portrayal of denial, she expresses her resolute devotion to her father. He is not moved by her love and sends her to her death. Feeling powerless to influence her fate, Iphigenia begins a process of dissociation. She is unable to come up with an argument that her life, independent of her father, is worth saving. She is worn down by manipulation and serves as currency in the male struggle for power. She willingly sacrifices herself. Helen, who has broken with patriarchy, lives, while

Iphigenia, who joins forces with it, dies. The motif of the father giving up or dismissing his daughter demonstrates how cut off men are from the feminine. Patriarchy constantly sends women the message that it is not safe for them unless they acquiesce and serve the needs of men and fall in line.

There are many images suggesting the nurse's body is not her own and that she is an object who belongs to others. The nurse in pornography serves the sexual needs of men. The pious nun is stripped of identity and duty-bound to pay attention only to the needs of others. It is difficult in a male-dominated culture to see deferential traits like subordination and sensitivity as strengths. Yet indeed the nurse's most striking attribute is her overriding responsiveness to others, which includes compliance with authority figures. She takes responsibility for others first. She may look confused, but she is processing information. Perceptive, she hears different points of view, evaluates, and acts on how best to serve. She does not judge. She is capable of understanding another perspective; that is true empathy.

Finding Voice

Voice connects what is on the inside to the outside. The silence and voicelessness of the nurse are displayed in *Miss Evers' Boys* and *The*

Nun's Story, which illustrate how such silence impacts healthcare. The nurse absorbs the patient's situation through constant verbal and non-verbal communication. She reports her assessment to physicians. She is often disregarded and dismissed. This unresolved conflict day after day wears her down and decreases her ability to trust what she has to say. It becomes easier to stay quiet in a messy situation than to step into it and voice her opinion. The audacity to speak one's mind falls away early in the nurse's career. Self-doubt settles in. She learns not to trust her knowledge, clinical acumen, and instincts. Instead she finds power through manipulation and covertness.

The nurse is not concerned with the idea of life but the fact of life. She has learned not to get hung up on emotions because she must be ready for the next crisis. She does not allow others to know her awkward and unpleasant feelings. She is inundated with intense emotions and favors outward distractions. Her soul is neglected. The soul wants its own intensity. As a society we fear depression but not nearly as much as we fear passion. Our culture teaches women to avoid disagreeing, making waves, and stewing. The nurse, by the nature of her role, remains compliant.

Filling the Void

We see the nurse's compulsive working as a way to prevent errors, and in a frenetic way, an attempt to control her chaotic environment. Yet we know something is wrong because of her exhaustion and tendency toward quick fixes for her own aches and pains. All of the additional tasks thrown at the nurse make it worse. Since she has no energy left for self reflection, creativity, and imagination, she focuses on working longer hours to fill the void. With so little time for herself, she seeks pleasure in unhealthy ways. She is diverted and influenced by advertisements that promise quick feel-good solutions. Consumer marketing exacerbates the confusion by telling the nurse what she should long for, which, in fact, pushes her true yearnings further away. Addictions supplant her inner wisdom and allow her to function in a highly rational and vigilant manner. Excess is a rebellion against perfection. She seeks to assert her right to be free. She is defiant against the inner and outer tyrant.

Compulsive behavior usually begins as an attempt to find spiritual meaning. Milk, honey, and grain, traditionally the foods of the goddess, are today's favorite foods in which to overindulge. It's as if the divine is speaking to the nurse spiritually through the allure of wine, reminding her of union through the yearning for sex, speaking of wisdom in the deep flavor of chocolate and coffee. These profane rituals have life-affirming sacred significance. Examples of overweight nurses are seen in *Misery*, *Romeo and Juliet*, and Dickens' character, Gamp. The desexualized matron is usually overweight. "Obesity is a manifestation of a soul that has more energy than the body can deal with," writes Marion Woodman. Perhaps this is a barrier against the anger and negative emotions of others.

Excess weight is also a barricade against impulses from within. Extra weight makes her stiff and inaccessible. Her largeness gives her power and serves as armor. C.G. Jung claims that, when primitive, infantile, and instinctual demands of the psyche are suppressed and pushed into the shadow, a split can occur, leading to substance abuse. Woodman theorizes that addictions arise when someone is looking for the nurturing and love they never received— a sort of primal bonding deficit.

We eat to affirm life. Food symbolizes the life force with which the body seeks to connect. It is common knowledge that food at the nurse's station disappears fast. With so much intensity, the nurse finds relief quickly in order to face it all again. Forget diet because that is more deprivation. Behavioral changes that rely on willpower do little long term. What she longs for is a way to express her imagination and sensitivity to counter the hierarchical demands. She accepts free dinners from pharmaceutical companies that give the illusion of living the high life while cluttering her life with worthless give-aways.

Even a motivated nurse tirelessly seeking new experiences comes up empty. It might be helpful to consciously view habits and automatic behavior as mysterious messages from the soul and become aware of them rather than attempt to change them. Instinctual or impulsive behavior actually shows an appetite and drive to live more fully. All nurses, on some level, are infantilized, patronized, harassed, or abused by the system or by those with whom they work. Spontaneity and joyous satisfaction disrupt the status quo. Finding her bigness and her power threatens the system that depends on invisible nurses. The most effective way to free the nurse is by replacing compulsiveness with pleasure. Once she knows what pleasure means deep within her soul, she can no longer be controlled by patriarchy.

Since the nurse has been trained in an Apollonian environment, she dismisses the Dionysian. Yet clearly she needs the moisture and appetite of Dionysus to be authentically in her body and do her best work. C.G. Jung argued that, since possession is part of the religious experience, and Christianity has excluded the lively, irrational Dionysian elements from ritual, we end up with addictions or possessions because we neglect the necessary experience. Dogma is no substitute for an inner religious experience. Many of my most profound spiritual experiences have come when opening my body in simple stretches, slowing down, and breathing.

Dipsomania, derived from the Greek words for *thirst* and *mania*, best describes the periodic acute craving for loosening by alcohol and what nurses experience when petitioned by Dionysus. It calls from the depths for intoxication to burn away monotony, certainty, and habit. The need for instant gratification is a signal that tolerance for anxiety is low. The nurse seeks quick solutions—pain medication, excess food, anti-anxiety drugs, and anti-depressants—which dull anxiety, as well as awareness. She may have skill and know how to look and sound good, but she is left with a profound emptiness. A false persona has no connection to the true self or authenticity. Drinking alcohol is an attempt to loosen constraints. Morally, this may be destructive, yet mythically, it is imperative.

Giving and Receiving

Giving is more comfortable than receiving and the nurse often has an inability to receive.

She fears dependency and denies that sometimes she is vulnerable. If the nurse was raised with conditional giving, she does not trust gifts and recognition, because, to her, there are always strings attached. Giving can also be about seeking approval and the illusion of love. If she accomplishes something, she downplays it. This behavior is seen again and again in Jackie when she brushes off praise. Receptivity, to the nurse, may be difficult and not feel safe if she has spent a lifetime protecting and defending herself. She may sacrifice anything to a man yet associates the word receptive with passivity and submission. However, being fully a woman, in creative work and in relationship, requires learning how to actively receive.

As we learn from myth, the union of Psyche and Eros produces a daughter, Pleasure, but this did not come about without trials and betrayal. I learned early in life how to channel emotional pain into my body. Physically, I was an athlete and chose sports requiring perfection like gymnastics and springboard diving. I knew how to listen to my body when I had an injury but I did not know how to find pleasure in my body. It wasn't until I understood the plight of Iphigenia that I was able to truly receive. Deep friendships, dreams, and mythology opened me. I could, although at first reluctantly, allow others to care for me in authentic and nonobligatory ways. A woman must willingly surrender and receive pleasure to experience her full potential.

Sadism and Masochism

The nurse is linked to the slave and the self-abnegating nun. Perhaps deep within the nurse, she carries a masochistic tendency. What is the allure of being abused, dominated, and mistreated? Romance and erotic novels have always carried the allure of the female being mastered by the male. There is something inherent in the female that finds being submissive and controlled erotic. The nurse also necessarily must have a bit of sadism. Her job includes injecting, inserting, and probing. Perhaps she releases repressed aggression by inflicting pain and controlling others.

The Invisible

Mythologically, the nurse operates under a veil, in the moonlight, and in darkness. She moves stealthily below the surface, a denizen of the underworld. She is often used as a disguise. For example, Hera and Demeter dressed as nurses to gain entrance into the human realm. The nurse uses her invisibility to her benefit. Much gets done under the radar. Belize, Jackie, and the unnamed nurse in *Romeo and Juliet* accomplish remarkable things without being noticed. They are insiders and there is a comfort in being undetectable.

The nurse and beggar recognize one another, both with street smarts, both from the ranks of the poor. The elderly nurse, Eurycleia, recognizes that the beggar is Odysseus when she catches sight of his scar. She knows him more intimately than his wife, Penelope, who doesn't identify him. The old crone is a common figure in mythology and folklore. Today she might be identified as the bag lady who reminds us of loneliness and insecurity—a survivor with peculiar wisdom, with no need for what the rest of society values. She is free yet scorned, but to most remains invisible.

Devouring Witch

The witch archetype has been rejected and twisted. She is a mean, controlling villain. The nurse uses this guise when she needs to scare visitors and keep them out of her space. The nurse works in a harsh and lonely place, often at night. She brings about altered states of consciousness. She possesses the power of prophecy. The word *witch* is associated with wit, meaning to perceive. The nurse's quick wit and humor reveal her personality. She has developed a level of insensitivity, in that she is, by necessity, numb. She can dissociate and split off from pain through various ways of anesthetizing herself. Witches live a disembodied existence, isolated from the community, desperately seeking to re-inhabit their body.

The mythological witch wants the vitality of youth and thus devours children as an attempt to embody them. Women deemed witches were real, living people. Midwives threatened church leaders the most because they had superior healing powers. In Neolithic times, the death-wielder is red, the color of life and fervor. The death lady has been degraded to scary witch or crooked old woman with a large nose. The vulture with broom-like wings, often associated with the witch, swoops down on corpses. The witch has no sword or armor, so she puts up an impenetrable barrier and cold demeanor to protect herself.

Envy

Envy, associated with the witch, is one of the most destructive emotions. In fact many murders are committed in the grip of envy. Talking about envy is taboo. It was heart-breaking for me to acknowledge its existence within the sisterhood of nursing. When I did, I entered a period of mourning. The nurse who envies wants to degrade and destroy what is good in another nurse since she cannot possess it herself. Hera is well known for envy. In one example, she disguises herself as a nurse and tricks Semele into destroying herself while pregnant with Dionysus. Envy within the sisterhood of nursing goes back to ancient times. I catalogued the many times I've been wounded by envy and the times I've watched it happen to others.

The victim of envy often reacts by deferring attention away from herself. She denies her unique qualities and tries to explain that she too has had a difficult life and things don't come easy for her. She feels guilty, takes responsibility for someone else's projections, and eventually withdraws, which brings more attacks from the envier. Her choices are to hold back or more fully let her talent shine. Nurses are careful not to stand out for fear that they will be ostracized. Envy among nurses maintains an expected status quo within the sisterhood.

The Backward Glance

The story of Orpheus and Eurydice illustrates how we cannot live in the past or possess another person. In patriarchy, the nurse is considered a possession, or sacrificial victim like Iphigenia, rather than a separate human being. As a condition of getting Eurydice out of the underworld, the only thing Orpheus must do is not look back until she reaches the surface. Fearful and overwhelmed by the potential loss of his possession, he cannot control this urge.

When he glances back, Hermes tells Eurydice he has done so, and she replies, "Who?" She has already forgotten him. He wants to live in the past and is unwilling to let her awaken and emerge as a separate person. In the myth, Eurydice stays in the underworld. Orpheus is dismembered by the maenads, symbolizing the truth that we cannot possess another person or live in the past.

Power

Most nurses are drawn to the profession by the desire to help others, yet the other side of the coin is power. The potential for abuse of power must be kept at a conscious level at all times. Nurses can intimidate, dominate, frighten, and potentially harm a patient, as demonstrated by Annie Wilkes. The nurse may lack the love she yearns for and cover it up with co-dependency. In the task-oriented hospital environment, she hides under statistics of success. The nurse experiences fear and anxiety when others hold power over her. She is kept from actual political power in the hierarchy because she is seen as dangerous and needing to be controlled. As women we are warned of the perils in pursuing power by the fate of figures in mythology, like Cassandra, Iphigenia, and Antigone.

Since nurses work in a power structure, they complain when they are not included in planning or policy making. Yet nurses tend to become indifferent when they are asked to sit on decision-making committees, seeing it as extra work and futile. They feel used by administrators who have their own agenda. I wonder about the root of this learned apathy. Does it come from the historical pattern of women being marginalized and obedient to authority?

Speaking up is often an investment of heart and soul. Self-preservation takes precedence as the nurse identifies with the role of supporter behind someone else's power. The powerful and the powerless work within an established set of customs, policies, and norms that keep the powerless exactly where they are. It is imperative that the nurse have a voice, not just for her benefit but for that of patients and healthcare.

In Favor of Melancholy and the Wilds

Melancholy used to be considered an affliction of the soul. Today it is labeled a disease—depression—to be treated with a pill rather than soul work. We don't take time for tragedy. Self-help books and short-term therapy perpetuate impatience. We do not go by the soul's clock, which requires time to backtrack, wander, saunter, feel, linger, and contemplate. The promise of a quick fix for things that have developed over a lifetime and through generations is self defeating.

What melancholy wants to teach us is wisdom, how to slow down, to feel life in its fullness, which includes the bittersweet, the sad, the romantic, and the passionate. Instead, we remain focused on progress and control, leaving little time to acknowledge our longings, stirrings, and tragedies. Melancholy is bigger than personal grief, loss or sadness. It is existential and carries the suffering of every human being. It carries our limitations, mortality, loss of innocence, and deepest regrets. Melancholy directs us down.

Melancholy wants attention—it is a symptom saying the soul has something to express. Melancholy used to be an accepted necessity to the creativity of poets, artists, blues singers, and philosophers. Melancholy speaks for the soul and does not want treatment. The word treatment has etymological roots in "to haul" or "to drag." Do we really want to haul or drag ourselves through life? We cannot mask what melancholy is trying to say.

We must determine what is missing. Passion, longing, and a tragic sensibility have much to teach. We label our passions disorders—unrequited love is equated with co-dependency and deep longings are labeled addictions. Appetite and intensity are not valued as enthusiasm and a zest for life. I am always horrified when someone dies tragically and people are quick to offer a reason. We blame the dead—"She didn't wear a seatbelt! He ate all the wrong things! She was an alcoholic, totally addicted!" Therefore, we look askance at tragedy. It is reduced to poor choices, somehow making those left behind feel better, further distanced from death.

The nurse, like Hecate, Hermes, Dionysus, and Baubo, is drawn to care for the maimed, vulnerable, odd, and down-and-out. There is an inherent wildness in her work. There is every kind of unpredictable bizarre situation and the nurse tolerates and even enjoys the abnormal, perverse, and aberrant. The deviant is unique and exciting. As in fairy tales, the nurse evokes surprise, wonder, awe, and admiration.

In addition to a high tolerance for the wild chaos of the hospital, the nurse still carries her acceptance of pain and humiliation, as seen in mythic figures like Ninshubur, Hygeia, and Dionysus, as well as in the film *The Nun's Story*. Freedom of choice is the essence of life. Since America has a recent history of enslavement, it is deep in our mythos and perhaps is played out in self-incarceration and self-sabotage. The blood of slaughtered Native Americans is in the soil where we live. What can we learn from their mythic capacity to slow down and listen?

THE SOUL OF THE NURSE

The soul longs to reveal its talents and hidden genius as well as its imperfect and defective features. Dreams are a good way to hear what the soul wants because waking life is too far removed from the unconscious.

Nurses have power in numbers, multifaceted knowledge, special skill, and public trust. Today's cultural value of individual autonomy is delusional in that it does not acknowledge the collective social need for the nurse and nursing care. The vast complexity of the nurse and the nature of the nursing experience itself is misunderstood and is not held with the deep respect, even reverence, as it ought to be. Why aren't nurses leaders in healthcare? The nurse will be even more powerful and helpful to society when she owns her own value system, not the one she is maladapted to, patriarchy's. We are informed by literature, art, and psychology, dominated by the male perspective. Even today, most of the psychology conferences have male speakers with a female audience. Women have begun to step up and tell their story, but it's just the beginning.

The nurse nourishes the weak, accepting the patient no matter what reckless neglect came before. The nurse is feared and desired and shows up when a person is injured, in need, or abandoned. She represents the impersonal relationship to fate and holds the fear evoked by illness, disfigurement, and hospitalization. She personifies the primal need for comfort, relief, and honesty. She is the gentle touch that restores life.

With her diffuse awareness, respect for others, reluctance to judge, concern for relationship, tolerance for complexity, and the Dionysian possibilities, the nurse holds much for society. If we continue to hide our individual and collective shadow, we remain unconscious to the soul. The nurse is obviously drawn to soul through her call to be a nurse. The word nurse derives from the Latin *nau*, associated with navigate, boat, ship, sailor, and the Latin *nutricius*, meaning nourishing. Like the depth-finder used to measure how deep the water is under a ship, the nurse helps navigate in and out of low points, on top of the unconscious, exploring the vast ocean without drowning. What about her soul? We know that for renewal she must accept her own vulnerability. Who is there to help her navigate, nourish her, and keep her from sinking and drowning?

CHAPTER 6

Re-membering the Soul of the Nurse

Unraveling the complexity of the nurse does not come without danger. Attempting to change long-held beliefs has consequences. Complicating matters, the nurse personifies what has been repressed for all women—her body, instincts, and natural desires. Accepting her true potential takes courage. How many of us want to face the enormity of this task? It is up to each nurse to make the shift within herself. Only then can nurses move collectively and begin to change the nursing culture.

The nurse's wisdom comes from her body. The fully embodied female is demanding that the nurse pay attention to her symptoms—depression, autoimmune diseases, addictions, weight problems, as well as the breakdown in the healthcare system. It is time to befriend the feminine in all her aspects because she is humanity's only hope.

Re-membering the soul of the nurse requires connecting to the nurse archetype. Since the nurse archetype is underground and seems invisible, we need to become aware of her split-off pieces. Each nurse can begin the process by connecting to her body and exploring her personal mythology, as I have done in this book. Acknowledging passion and pleasure, following the examples of Dionysian maenads and Aphrodite, leads to nurse empowerment.

The nurse's unique vocation allows her to enter into ritual in her everyday work. This can be as simple as recognizing hand washing, giving report, and drawing up medication as ritual. On a psychological level, it is essential that nurses no longer sacrifice their own authority solely for the profits and ambitions of others. It is time to move from daughter to full womanhood.

The nurse participates in ritual every day. Ritual deepens meaning and commitment to the profession as well as honoring its ancestry. The nurse ebbs and flows with the reality of constant change, loss, finitude, and the miraculous rebounding of the human body and spirit. She tends her patient, not at a distance, but up close. The nurse, connected to her own darkness, wetness, and earthy nature, is aligned with the source of her true power. Like mythic Vesta, who attends to the home and hearth, the nurse tends the public fire. She carries illumination. Her connection to the body and earth is not sterile. She must be connected to her body to do her best work.

If we continue to see the nurse as inferior or on the margins, we need a new paradigm that sheds light on its merits. The nurse thrives on the margins. It is not a matter of moving away but toward these exiled borders. Collectively the nurse has humble roots and her work is absolutely unpretentious. The word humiliation is derived from *humus* which has to do with the earth. It is also closely associated with humid and wet. To be humiliated is to be brought down to earth, into wetness and decomposition. Perhaps this is why nurses tolerate humiliation so well. Nurses grasp the bigger picture and intuitively understand their rootedness in the earth. When the nurse can get her arms around humiliation mythologically, she can move out of the repetitive pattern of helplessness. Rather than deny or suppress what it means to be humble, she can integrate it and move forward.

The Paradox of Silence

The inner sense of connection with others is essential to the nurse. Rather than risk open conflict or disagreement that might lead to disconnection, nurses remain silent. Attending the patient with a touch, a smile, or a gesture, the nurse communicates significant messages without words. Physicians are typically in a hurry, rarely in silent communication with patients. For communion, the patient relies on the nurse. The nurse also knows that forced sharing can be destructive. Nurses learn quickly that it's best for patients to share only when they are ready. Silence is necessary for internal clarity and grounding.

As a young girl, I worked cattle with my father who was a man of few words. It was up to me to learn by observation. As we drove to the ranch, I'd ask him what we were going to do that day and he'd grin and turn up the classical music on the radio. On the ranch, he communicated with me from across the field with a simple look, hand movement, shout, or gesture. I learned how to ride a horse, gather cattle, brand, and vaccinate through observation. Nightingale claimed observation is the most important attribute of the nurse. We are reminded of its significance through mythic figures such as Ninshubur and Hygeia, as well as Gabrielle in *The Nun's Story*.

Some nurses are bottled up and unable to express themselves. They find their rage surfacing as irritability, sabotage between nurses, or depression. That's why it's so important for the nurse to be exquisitely in touch with her body. Sensations of the body are essential indicators to observe, such as a clenched jaw or upset stomach. Finding ways to unlock emotions held in the body are actually critical to health, especially in a stressful occupation like nursing. Women's rage is often rooted in feelings of abandonment, betrayal, and rejection, both personally and collectively.

Body language is very important. Social psychologists agree that two-thirds of communication is done without words. Nurses are conditioned to be pleasant, even smile, when communicating crucial information. Unfortunately, when a nurse smiles, she might not be taken seriously. Finding the authentic inner voice requires excavation. Each nurse must find a way to express herself, especially her inner stirrings. She must mourn her losses and consider actions that are authentically hers, not simply imitate someone else.

Not long ago I felt grounded in this way when I stood to make a comment in a large audience of psychotherapists. After I spoke, people came up and told me what I said resonated for them. In the past I'd felt intimidated, my heart pounding and hands sweating, so I'd stay in my seat. The year before, I'd had a thyroidectomy for a carcinoma secondary to the radiation treatment I had when I was a teenager. Typically I avoid surgeons. Like most nurses, I give them a wide path. So I was surprised when an incredible advocacy developed between my surgeon and me. But first I had to earn his respect.

I had a good surgical experience and follow-up with this highly skilled surgeon. Later I was angry about something and needed to tell him. I practiced exactly what I wanted to say, looking at myself in a mirror with specific attention not to smile or give over to my predisposition to please. When we met, I did the same thing and he got it. He has listened to me attentively ever since.

Removing my thyroid freed my voice. I have since shared with him the part he played in my symbolic and mythological process. Something needed to be cut out. After surgery it was a new voice, one that connected to the earth. It came through my feet, up through my body, and exited in my breath from the portal of my throat. Our life experiences give each of us these kinds of opportunities, yet they are not always easy to recognize.

Jung claimed that an unconscious secret is more injurious than a conscious one. Most secrets within the sisterhood of nursing are conscious. Secrets are important because they differentiate us from the rest of the community. There is so much complexity and generational knowledge in what the nurse actually does that it makes little sense to try to explain much of it—just like the gallows humor that keeps nurses sane but would horrify others. This is why we know so little about ancient rites, rituals, and clandestine organizations. Secrets are important in maintaining a sacred covenant among those who understand and have earned it. The nurse-patient relationship is confidential, thus considered a secret. Secrets involve a compelling paradox because confessing one's innermost secrets is cathartic and cleansing.

Sometimes illness uncovers secrets the body has kept safely locked away. This is illustrated in *The English Patient*. Secrets can be felt in the body even when all evidence suggests transparency. We feel something is untrue in our body, yet we deny our instincts, perceptions, and feelings. When secrets are discovered, it can be quite painful and leave us feeling betrayed. Some believe getting over betrayal is about forgiveness. The tendency to tolerate appalling behavior and be quick to forgive is frequently seen in the public realm.

Robin Morgan, author and leader in the women's movement, asserted that radical feminist Andrea Dworkin, after horrific abuse by her former husband, was still "reaching out to understand him, still comprehending his motivation, his despair, more than her own." Similarly, in August 2012, successful pop singer Rihanna confessed in a tearful television interview that she had been protective of boyfriend, Chris Brown, after he beat her. She was worried that public criticism would keep him from getting the help he needed.

To me, forgiveness and compassion come too easily and often lead to more betrayal. Forgiveness is too closely linked to dogma. An honest reconciliation can take place only when both parties are equally invested. Acceptance, however, of the way things are, owning up, and taking responsibility for our part are key to getting unstuck. We cannot change others.

Abandonment as Gift

The mythology of the orphan has much to tell us. Yet, because our culture tends toward possessing one another, it's difficult to take in the positive, freeing aspect of being orphaned. Instead, we cling to our heartbreak and sense of being deserted. In Greek mythology, Ariadne becomes the beloved of Dionysus only after she is abandoned, mourns, finds her inner strength, and accepts that she is truly alone. Abandonment, betrayal, and being orphaned actually offer liberation from suffocating roles and bestow spiritual freedom.

I've found that only when I accept that I've been betrayed can I move beyond anger. When I stop trying to figure out the motives of the other person, as if he or she sees the world as I do, I can let go of the illusions I've held dear. My best friendships have always developed when I was most alone. In my experience, human relationships are based on our flaws—what is weak, helpless, and in need. By showing our vulnerabilities, we are seen clearly for who we are.

We must also come to terms with the unconscious devouring aspect within us that wants to catch, own, and imprison others. Perhaps this explains something about why the veteran nurse sometimes eats the young nurse. We all long to feed off that which is full of life, vigorous, and innocent. I think about my own experience as I entered my midlife sexual renaissance and became playfully attracted to a friend's son in his mid-twenties. We joked about my name, Mrs. Robinson, and had a lot of fun with it. However, when I looked at it mythologically, I was fantasizing about the innocent, vital, untapped potential within him as I faced moving into midlife with my own loss of purity and innocence. It's taboo, even today, to speak of such a thing for a woman, yet it is a common practice for a middle-aged man to leave his wife for a much younger woman. Only by living within ambiguity, where repulsion and attraction meet, are we whole. Dionysian consciousness breaks boundaries and expands how we see things.

Sacred Instincts

The Dionysian maenad does not make a sacrifice—she is the sacrifice. She symbolizes the torture of not being remembered and calls the soul to vulnerability and woundedness. She must enter the underworld. Her new life emerges from the abyss. Once the nurse learns how to receive, she can sacrifice to pleasure without guilt or fear of too much joy. She can go deeper, connecting with eros, her body, and her feminine soul. In Ancient Greece there were ecstatic festivals of initiation. With no outlet today, facing the depths often feels like madness. A terror comes over us when we even begin to think of letting go. Our coping strategies have kept our demons at bay. Without relationship to the wild, we go wild in our psyche or turn to compulsions. The maenad is totally given over to the dark. Dionysus will receive her only when she sacrifices herself completely. Symbolically the maenad temporarily surrenders her persona as nurse. Receptivity must be learned away from the Apollonian environment.

Some time ago, following my instincts, I left the central valley and a well paid CNS job. It was time to move to the ocean where my maternal ancestors once lived. I hungered to study, to write, and to get in touch with my body. I wanted to dive into my research on the nurse. I gave up my large house and material possessions that would not fit in the tiny rented cottage. I had to let go of stagnant attitudes and relationships. The deaths of my parents catapulted me into my new hometown where the dolphins can be seen swimming off shore. The cottage I share with my husband is probably 100 years old. Despite its mere 600 square feet, lack of water pressure, and inadequate electrical outlets, I need nothing.

Archetypal experiences can produce euphoric openings as well as dramatic humiliations. I abandoned myself to the experience, submitted, and received. Dionysus became my teacher in breaking with convention as he evoked the maenad within me. Western medicine has been, and continues to be, a big part of my personal and professional life. But I knew early in my life that I could not fully recover from physical illness without tending my soul.

The nurse understands madness. Her job is to be sane in a mad world. Her Dionysian sensibilities equip her with the ability to integrate what has been censured and suppressed. Why does she neglect her own body? Does she associate all bodies with messy disfigurement and decay? Nothing disgusts Dionysus. It is Apollo who seeks clean, refined aesthetics and sterile rooms. Dionysus accepts the generative slime of nature—bleeding, birthing, sweating, fat, body hair, aging, and death. Like Nightingale, the maenad nurse is desperate for depth over superficiality because she knows death and re-birth are necessary for regeneration.

THE SOUL OF THE NURSE

What would a festival of initiation look like for nurses? The frescoes at the Villa of Pompeii show maenads giving over to their instinctual longings, lowering their inhibitions with wine. They symbolically pass through the body of a woman in an initiation ritual of rebirth. Today female initiation happens mostly alone, accessing heart through solitary practice.

Those unwilling to work with shadow can't understand why their life isn't working. Rather than accept the contribution they are making to the havoc, they plead victim and create further illusions to block reality. It's difficult to admit to oneself what is weak and broken. We can learn to pull a projection back only by acknowledging it. By accepting the shameful parts of ourselves, we embrace not only our complexity but our entire being. The nurse who avoids self-reflection will eventually tire of agitation, burn out, or be undone by her tears when she looks in the mirror. It's never too late to move toward consciousness.

There are many folklore motifs depicting the nurse as a helpful animal. Animal nature includes body, sex, and aggression. Women are taught at an early age to suppress their animal nature in order to avoid being ostracized. Since the nurse is often portrayed as sex object, she can have fun with it. It's important for nurses to fully embrace their instincts and desires.

Eroticism is the natural conduit to feminine maturity. When the nurse sacrifices to pleasure and embraces the ambiguity of her sexuality, she is fully empowered.

The Ambiguity of Pleasure

Since the nurse requires strict discipline in her practice, it often spills over into the rest of her life. Key to pleasure is spontaneity, which, for most nurses, means facing her perfectionism and compulsions. Punishing her body, as nurses routinely do with long shifts and intense work, maintains the split, as do rigid schedules that prevent unplanned activities. Discipline holds, for most, a negative connotation, but we all know that no nurse completes her training or passes the board exam without it. Another way to look at it is that the word *discipline* is linked to disciple or pupil. The pupil who loves the teacher is enthusiastic, open to new ideas, and receptive. The female orgasm takes a disciplined and determined effort for most women. Speaking as a heterosexual, my generation and those before were taught that it was up to the man to give the woman pleasure. A male partner can help support a woman's orgasm but ultimately it is up to her. It takes discipline, a determined beginner's mind, and love between pupil and teacher—soul and body.

With this in mind, a woman enjoying the pleasure of her body is highly suppressed and taboo. For example, in 2012, a nun and Yale scholar, Sister Margaret Farley, ignited controversy with her book, *Just Love: A Framework for Christian Sexual Ethics* (2006), with her statement that masturbation does no harm and actually helps women discover their own pleasure and enhances relationships. The Vatican labels masturbation "an intrinsically and gravely disordered action." Farley received harsh criticism and censure by the Vatican. In a related incident in 1994, Surgeon General Joycelyn Elders was asked at a United Nations AIDS conference whether masturbation ought to be taught as a means of preventing riskier sexual activity. She replied, "I think it is part of human sexuality, and perhaps it should be taught." She was fired. These are just two examples of the fear and hypocrisy women face regarding pleasure and sexuality. Women cannot even talk about masturbation publicly without serious repercussions.

In another incident in 2012, Columbia law student Sandra Fluke was vilified and called a slut after testifying before the House of Representatives in favor of insurance coverage for birth control. Opinions against such coverage came from the panel of all-male priests and ministers. Under these abysmal conditions, each woman must remember that physical pleasure, represented by Aphrodite, is always associated with vitality and love and is not a marker of a bad woman. The oppression of Aphrodite has found its way into our culture through advertising and pornography. Scholars avoid discussing Aphrodite, finding her the most alarming of the twelve Olympians, even though archeological evidence suggests she is the most important.

Aphrodite

Aphrodite's desire goes beyond lust. There is reverence for beauty, pleasure, and grace, as she is the counter-force to harsh realities and pain. Aphrodite expresses sensuality and the ability to give and receive pleasure and joy. She attracts, connects, and binds to nature through the body. For a woman, sacred moments come from moving more deeply into her body. The nurse loses sight of her inner Aphrodite when she identifies exclusively with media and advertising. Images that are airbrushed and photoshopped only succeed in making natural imperfections contemptible.

In opposition to Aphrodite, our relatedness is now maintained less in person and more on electronic devices. I am always horrified when I see people, out together, spending more time looking at their tiny, handheld screens than connecting with one another. There seems to be terror associated with satisfying our natural proclivity for direct human contact. Paradoxically, through the Internet, women are now connecting with one another as modern-day servants to Aphrodite, teaching and guiding one another in the ways of pleasure, beauty, and fleshly union. As the nurse moves into her relationship with pleasure, she liberates her sensual and spiritual potential. When she knows what pleasure means and feels it deeply in her body, she can no longer be controlled by patriarchy.

The Ambiguity of the Female Body

Eighteen months before his death, I attended a James Hillman conference. He spent the last morning talking about the nurse and asked if there were any nurses in the audience. Knowing Hillman's history of berating anyone that dared speak from the audience, I did not raise my hand. A few other nurses did and were predictably shot down.

Despite Hillman's well-known brash treatment of his audience, I have always resonated with his writings and have found his material to be provocative and life-changing. Perhaps growing up with so many arrogant brothers and working so many years with self-important physicians has conditioned me to be able to spot and appreciate a brilliant mind, no matter the persona.

The image Hillman brought up was *The Roman Charity*, which started to show up in fresco paintings 2000 years ago and continues to appear, as in the last scene of John Steinbeck's *Grapes of Wrath*. The image depicts a young nurse breastfeeding an old man. The story behind the image describes a daughter breastfeeding her father, who has been incarcerated and sentenced to death by starvation. Some claim the actual first telling of the story portrays a daughter breastfeeding her mother. If this story had endured, maybe the mother-daughter immortality mystery, that shows they are one, would have continued to dominate our culture.

Hillman explained that the image, absolutely archetypally accurate, is the correct role for the nurse because in the image she ensures the future of the old man's soul. The women in the audience were furious yet had difficulty saying why. It was a lively few hours. The thing I appreciate most about Hillman is his ability to explain opposite ends of any concept. As soon as you think you get it, he presents the counter-view and you somehow get that too. It is very uncomfortable yet challenging and therefore enriching. However, he is not a woman. Hillman seemed enamored with the virgin-maiden qualities of the nurse yet played down the darker and erotic side. A lactating nurse has been pregnant, thus cannot be a virgin-maiden. She is a sexually active woman.

The feminine has been reduced in so many ways in the service of men—beauty, support, obedience—her worth dependent on men's desires and needs. So I continued to try to understand the image symbolically from the nurse's perspective. The image reflects the natural and mythological truth that no one survives without the feminine, without the nurse. There is no doubt that the nurse influences, educates, and transforms through her body. Each of us has a thirst for nurturance, protection, and human kindness.

I have always had a soft place in my heart for old men and, mythologically, the young daughter is naturally drawn to the old man, like Cordelia to King Lear, Antigone to Oedipus, and Iphigenia to Agamemnon. By being nursed by the young woman, the old man stays alive and helps her integrate her inner authority through logic, judgment, and counsel. She feels seen by the old man. He has few needs. Their language is sweet and feels safe. He gets her, does not criticize her, does not tease her, and makes her feel good. He represents love without judgment.

There is great reward for the nurse when she makes another feel better. Perhaps *The*

Roman Charity is the ultimate symbolic gesture—the full surrender and giving of her own body to another body while integrating her own masculine, breaking free of mores and succumbing to true feminine power. The image shows the power she has over others to feed or not to feed from her body.

The Roman Charity is not simply a pious act of obligation to feed someone in need, nor is it a pornographic distortion in which the woman's body exists for the use of men. We see in this image that the nurse is a Dionysian maenad, letting down her milk and letting go of civilizing aspects, deepening her connection with nature. We see this not only in the nurse's gesture but also in the old man who surrenders. He is soft, not pushing, and has given over to his vulnerability and is receiving. It is an act of choice for the nurse yet the stimulus is instinctual.

We are born of woman, fed from her placenta, then her breasts, and, when we are old and ill, we need her to survive, ultimately turning toward her in death. Humanity's only hope is to realize its dependence on the lactating capacity of woman. Something a man can never have. The prerequisite of renewal is acceptance of dependency and need. Perhaps this is why *The Roman Charity* holds such a healing image of renewal. The nurse is holding and tending the soul of the old man so it can go forward. The old dying man accepts his dependency and surrenders his patriarchal power to the nurse.

From Daughter to Full Womanhood

To move into full womanhood, the nurse needs connection to her original source. The feminine teaches us how to accept our vulnerabilities, live in the now, and leave the past behind. Both genders acquire this capacity from their feminine side although, unless the nurse claims her inner masculine as well, nothing will change. Only then does she stand in her own inner authority.

Death does not end a relationship. The inner father and mother live on in the psyche. Destructive patterns continue. The nurse who continues to project her inner father outwardly remains bound to patriarchy that does not value the significance of the feminine. Each daughter must acknowledge her father's shadow and come to terms with his rage, arrogance, denial, selfishness, and greed. I idealized my father. Exposing this illusion empowered me because it allowed me to integrate my own masculine traits. Only when I accepted the true humanness and fallibilities of my father did I begin the move into my own authority, shed the role of daughter, and retrieve the valuable feminine that is rightly mine.

The nurse need not continue to collude with patriarchy. She can pull projections back from physicians and institutions when she owns that part of herself. Each nurse must step out of her comfort zone and risk being an outcast. As Rollo May puts it, "Every human being must have a point at which [s]he stands against the culture, where [s]he says, this is me and the damned world can go to hell." Encouraging eccentricities can actually improve our professional life. Women in the past have been far more courageous. As long as the nurse looks outside herself for fulfillment she will be unfamiliar with her inner wisdom. She must give up her fantasy that patriarchy will fulfill her needs. She must provide for and protect herself.

When the nurse is not connected to her body, she loses contact with her most essential resource, her inner life of dreams and imagination. I've experienced an odd sort of fear when making connections in my writing. Something comes over me that makes me want to stop writing and find a distraction. It is as if my psyche can't accommodate all the ideas coming through me. I've come to the conclusion that personal identity needs to be strong enough to contain the creative flow. It is not my rational ego mind doing the creating. It is coming from a deeper source. The stronger the personal identity, the more flexible it becomes. If the nurse's ego is strong, she will trust her instincts and inner wisdom. Women feel deeply through their body in dance, yoga, an embrace, breastfeeding, making love, or being with another during birth or death. Jung and Nightingale made similar claims and believed the body and spirit are one.

Physicians and nurses have very different skills, sensibilities, and wisdom. The Apollonian focus of clarity, control, distance, and separate autonomy is necessary. The Dionysian merges and collaborates with the murky and mysterious ways in which life actually plays out. Objectivity and distance shield one from human relationships while the intensity of these relationships is the essence of nursing. Both are crucial.

Some Thoughts on Sisterhood

I spent a week at Esalen in Big Sur last year at a women's retreat that culminated in an evening of soaking in private natural hot tubs overlooking the Pacific Ocean. I felt joyful, like Persephone when she was a young maiden with her girlfriends. We prepared all day, picking fresh herbs and flowers from the grounds and seaweed from the ocean, to make the tubs fragrant. Candles illuminated the room. We sang songs and took turns floating one another in the water. We gave and received massages and sugar scrubs. That week with women—of secret baths and rituals––affected me deeply, grounding me in my body and bonding me to my new sisters. Ritual is like a web that protects and catches us when we fall. Pleasure, sensuality, sharing stories and wisdom can uncover the mythos connecting the nurse to her body and nature.

My experience occurred away from home and the work setting. All nurses need these experiences, yet we need not postpone them due to the belief that we have to go to a far-off spiritual land or create a new healing temple for ritual. We can experience profound sacred ritual wherever we are, even in our daily routines. Aphrodite is sorely missed today in nursing. A sisterhood between nurses has the potential to create a sacred trust based on a solid ancestral and mythological foundation. We do not need to re-create the ancient women's mysteries. As we open our hearts to new possibilities, our true nurse image will emerge with the reverence it deserves.

The Soul of the Nurse

As a young ambitious woman raised among men I needed to learn the ways of womanhood. I went to nursing school because I loved science, psychology, and connecting on a deep personal level with people. In nursing school, I absorbed every detail of the sciences, as well as how to give a bath or a back rub, make a bed, serve a food tray, and feed a patient. It was my introduction to nurturing. Perhaps other nurses, like me, went to nursing school to learn how to be a nurturer, wanting it for themselves but never quite having found it, thus attempting to make a career out of nurturing and protecting others.

Not long ago I was lying in *savasana*, the corpse pose, at the end of a restorative yoga class on the anniversary of my mother's death. Hearing the teacher's gentle voice, I slowed down and felt the teacher's soft loving touch on my body. Locked emotions surfaced. As I surrendered to these unexpected emotions, I realized that the anxious, fast-paced, busy, non-tender part of my mother in me could die. I could open my heart, receive love, and listen to my body. The point of feminine consciousness is not to resolve matter into spirit, but to hold the tension of opposites, to perceive spirit and matter as one. This type of perception is not possible in strictly Apollonian and masculine consciousness.

Mythology speaks to the unconscious. What we learn from Orpheus' backward glance is that we cannot relive the past. The goal is not to repeat. Tears of melancholy add moisture to the soul. Dry humor or a raw wit offers an angry person release and access to a soul overflowing with tears. Symptoms arise when we unconsciously ignore our destiny.

The final week of editing this book took me to the Ojai valley during a heat wave with no air conditioning. It was like the town in the central valley where I grew up. The flat-roofed house had an uncanny resemblance to the house where I was raised. There were orchards and roses, cotton-tail bunnies, and quail. On Friday night, a nearby high school football game interrupted my silence with a band and loud cheering. Without television, music, or any of my usual distractions, memories of childhood flooded over me as I read the manuscript one last time. I was dismembered once again. Once the nurse knows she has a calling, she cannot betray it. She chooses nursing out of necessity. She is called by a greater force.

Poet Jack Hirschman puts it this way, "Go to your broken heart. If you don't have one, get one." Seven years ago, my parents died, less than six months apart, and quickly the illusion of my family fell apart in a rapid succession of heartbreaking scenarios. It was a time of complete confusion which shook me to my core and broke me into many pieces. At the time, a friend pierced my heart when she said that my ordeal was simply a chapter in my story. I replied, "Yes, one day I am sure it will be, but not now." I knew I needed to suffer and mourn. Mourning is necessary to move from youth to maturity. Life is both fair and unfair. Betrayals and subsequent grieving nudged me forward. It was my soul that refused to die and insisted I take the time and attention to re-member and put the pieces back together again in a new way. I have begun to understand the term *amor fati*— love of one's fate. My orphaned soul always wanted to push out and expand beyond my upbringing.

Each nurse is unique, valuable, and imperfect, with mysterious complexities. Within the sisterhood of nursing, the essence of the nurse is acknowledged and understood. Each nurse has her own particularities yet she is grounded in the archetype. It is time to re-vision ourselves and fulfill the unfinished business of our ancestors. Imagination opens to vocation.

PRAISE FOR *THE SOUL OF THE NURSE*

"*The Soul of the Nurse* is a unique work. It is an inspiring exploration of the mythology and archetypal foundations that empower the deepest healing instincts of the nursing profession. This level of understanding is essential for any profession, if it is to achieve its highest possibilities. Robinson has performed a valuable service for nursing. May it spread to other professions as well!"

> Larry Dossey, MD
> Author: *Reinventing Medicine and The Power of Premonitions*
> *Executive Editor: Explore: The Journal of Science and Healing*

"As an experienced Critical Care Nurse, Elizabeth Robinson–first hand–has lived and witnessed the various enigmatic aspects of nursing. In her groundbreaking book, *The Soul of the Nurse*, she unveils the many mysteries of the nurse in a way we can all easily comprehend, embrace and be touched by. This homage to a very special group of healers honors and shines light on their journey. I highly recommend this book to anyone in the nursing or healthcare profession."

> Cheri Clampett, ERYT
> Co-author: *The Therapeutic Yoga Kit*

"*The Soul of the Nurse* is a valuable addition to the literature of nursing. It will help nurses find their voice and step into their power in these chaotic times in healthcare. This book is also an important social contribution, because no society can flourish without the essential contributions of nurses."

> Barbara Montgomery Dossey, PhD, RN, FAAN
> Author: *Florence Nightingale: Mystic, Visionary,*
> *Healer and Holistic Nursing*

"What Joseph Campbell did to explain myth, Elizabeth Robinson does for nursing. She reveals the inner meanings of the nurse's role to revitalize an essential profession. The revolutionary insights in *The Soul of the Nurse* offer renewal to those at the center of healthcare."

> Jonathan Young, PhD Psychologist
> *Founding Curator, Joseph Campbell Archives*